Milady's Standard Professional Barbering Exam Review

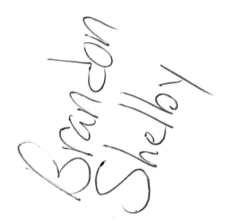

CENGAGE
Learning™

Australia • Brazil • Japan • Korea • Mexico • Singapore • Spain • United Kingdom • United States

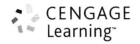
CENGAGE
Learning™

**MILADY'S STANDARD
Professional Barbering Exam
Review, Fifth Edition**
Milady

President, Milady: Dawn Gerrain

Publisher: Erin O'Connor

Acquisitions Editor:
Martine Edwards

Product Manager:
Jessica Mahoney

Editorial Assistant: Maria Hebert

Director of Beauty Industry
Relations: Sandra Bruce

Senior Marketing Manager:
Gerard McAvey

Production Director:
Wendy Troeger

Senior Content Project
Manager: Nina Tucciarelli

Senior Art Director: Joy Kocsis

For product information and
technology assistance, contact us at **Professional & Career
Group Customer Support, 1-800-648-7450**

For permission to use material from this text or product,
submit all requests online at **cengage.com/permissions**
Further permissions questions can be emailed to
permissionrequest@cengage.com

Library of Congress Control Number: 2010926975

ISBN-13: 978-1-4354-9712-2

ISBN-10: 1-4354-9712-0

Milady
5 Maxwell Drive
Clifton Park, NY 12065-2919
USA

Cengage Learning products are represented in Canada by
Nelson Education, Ltd.

For your lifelong learning solutions, visit **milady.cengage.com**

Visit our corporate website at **cengage.com**

Printed in the United States of America
1 2 3 4 5 XX 14 13 12 11 10

Milady's Standard
Professional Barbering Exam Review

Foreword v

PART I—CHAPTER REVIEW TESTS 1

CHAPTER 1—Study Skills 1

CHAPTER 2—The History of Barbering 4

CHAPTER 3—Professional Image 7

CHAPTER 4—Microbiology 11

CHAPTER 5—Infection Control and Safe Work Practices 15

CHAPTER 6—Implements, Tools, and Equipment 22

CHAPTER 7—Anatomy and Physiology 28

CHAPTER 8—Chemistry 36

CHAPTER 9—Electricity and Light Therapy 42

CHAPTER 10—Properties and Disorders of the Skin 46

CHAPTER 11—Properties and Disorders of the Hair and Scalp 53

CHAPTER 12—Treatment of the Hair and Scalp 61

CHAPTER 13—Men's Facial Massage and Treatments 64

CHAPTER 14—Shaving and Facial Hair Design 73

CHAPTER 15—Men's Haircutting and Styling 79

CHAPTER 16—Men's Hair Replacement 88

CHAPTER 17—Women's Haircutting and Styling 92

CHAPTER 18—Chemical Texture Services 96

CHAPTER 19—Haircoloring and Lightening 105

CHAPTER 20—Nails and Manicuring 113

CHAPTER 21—State Board Preparation and Licensing Laws 117

CHAPTER 22—The Job Search 120

CHAPTER 23—Barbershop Management 123

PART II—SAMPLE STATE BOARD EXAMINATIONS. **127**

Sample State Board Examination Test 1 127

Sample State Board Examination Test 2 143

Sample State Board Examination Test 3 159

Answers to Chapter Review Tests **175**

Answers to Sample State Board Examinations **183**

PART III—HELPFUL REMINDERS FOR EXAMINATION DAY **186**

Foreword

The purpose of this book is to assist barbering students in their preparation for state board examinations. The contents of this book mirror the changes and updates reflected in the 5th edition of *Milady's Standard Professional Barbering* textbook and serve to provide examination candidates with an overall review of the material therein. This material review is presented in a multiple-choice test format, which represents the standard examination form adopted by the majority of state barber boards for written and computer-based examinations.

Part I, Chapter Review Tests, provides a comprehensive review test for each textbook chapter. These tests are designed to provide a detailed review of the subject matter found in each chapter and should be used by students to evaluate their personal level of understanding in a specific subject area. Students will then be able to identify subject areas in which they have a clear understanding and those areas that need additional review or study prior to completing the Sample State Board Examinations in Part II.

In Part II, three Sample State Board Examinations have been compiled from the chapter review tests. Each subject area is represented by several questions, of the most universally relevant questions for that topic and its application to the field of barbering, that may be included in a state board examination.

It is recommended that instructors review the questions in each 150-item test to determine the relevancy of the question topics to their particular state board exams. For example, some states may not require testing in nail histology or manicuring because the subject is not included in the barbering curriculum. Other states may not require testing in chemical services applications. Therefore it becomes the responsibility of barber instructors to provide students with *specific* guidance regarding the state board examination in their state.

Part III, Helpful Reminders for Examination Day, provides a general guideline for exam candidates to follow when preparing for written or computer-based and practical examinations. It is recommended that instructors review these guidelines as well, adapt the information to conform with the procedures of their state barber board, and share the results with their students.

PART I—Chapter Review Tests

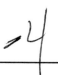

CHAPTER 1—STUDY SKILLS

Multiple Choice

1. Which type of students will not benefit as much as others from a review of study skills?
   a. Students in their second or third postsecondary educational experience
   b. Students in preparation for a second career
   c. Students returning to barbering after a brief absence
   d. Students who studied barbering as undergraduates   _A_

2. A sense of _____ toward your studies will help you understand and apply what is taught.
   a. discipline   c. entitlement
   b. adventure   d. None of the answers are correct.   _A_

3. It is a good idea to keep _____ organized in a tote bag for easy storage or transfer to the classroom.
   a. books   c. supplies
   b. paper   d. All answers are correct.   _D_ C

4. Writing the information down is a method of _____.
   a. building long-term memory   c. repetition
   b. acronyms   d. mnemonics   _A_ d

5. To enhance your _____, try categorizing the information into smaller segments.
   a. long-term memory   c. study skills
   b. short-term memory   d. barbering skills   _A_ b

6. To promote better _____, try to associate new information with prior knowledge through word association techniques.
   a. long-term memory   c. repetition
   b. short-term memory   d. acronyms   _D_ a

7. A mind map is not a _____.
   a. helpful study skill   c. mnemonic
   b. note taking technique   d. method for building connections   _C_

8. SHAPES is a(n) _____ for the functions of the skin: sensation, heat regulation, absorption, protection, excretion, and secretion.
    a. acronym
    b. rhyme
    c. mind map
    d. None of the answers are correct.

    A

9. When mind-mapping, subconnections are created _____.
    a. first
    b. second
    c. last
    d. None of the answers are correct.

    D

10. The _____ of an outline should be the topic or concept to be covered.
    a. subject
    b. title
    c. subcategory
    d. acronym

    B

11. In an outline, B identifies the _____.
    a. first main topic
    b. second main topic
    c. first subtopic
    d. second subtopic

    D

12. _____ takes place during the planning step of writing a paper.
    a. Brainstorming
    b. Editing
    c. Outlining
    d. Revising

    A

13. During the drafting stage of writing a paper, _____ takes place.
    a. brainstorming
    b. formal outlining
    c. note-taking
    d. editing

    B

14. _____ occurs during the revising stage of writing a report.
    a. Brainstorming
    b. Research
    c. Rewriting
    d. Proofreading

    C

15. During the editing stage of writing a paper, you should _____.
    a. create an outline
    b. brainstorm
    c. take notes
    d. check punctuation

    D

16. The four distinct learning styles are combinations of _____.
    a. two emotional styles and two physical styles
    b. two ways of perceiving and two ways of processing
    c. four different memory techniques
    d. None of the answers are correct.

    B

17. Another name for dynamic learners is _____ learners.
    a. intuitive   c. movement-based
    b. common-sense   d. quick   A

18. "What?" is the _____ learner's favorite question.
    a. dynamic   c. analytic
    b. common-sense   d. innovative   C

19. If you feel particularly energetic after dinner, your best study time would be _____.
    a. 8 am   c. 2 pm
    b. 10 am   d. 8 pm   D

CHAPTER 2—THE HISTORY OF BARBERING

Multiple Choice

1. All of the following statements about early barbering practitioners are true except that they _____.
    - a. were shamans or priests in some cultures
    - b. were held in high esteem
    - c. were held in low esteem
    - d. used tools made from flints   _____

2. According to archaeological studies, animal sinews _____.
    - a. were not used for haircare
    - b. were avoided by shamans and medicine men
    - c. were used to tie the hair back
    - d. were used as haircutting implements   _____

3. The Latin word *tonsorial* means the cutting, clipping, or trimming of hair with _____.
    - a. only shears
    - b. only a razor
    - c. shears or a razor
    - d. None of the answers are correct.   _____

4. Some tribes believed that cutting the hair _____.
    - a. exorcised bad spirits
    - b. served as a sacrifice to the gods
    - c. brought good spirits
    - d. None of the answers are correct.   _____

5. In Egyptian culture, the hair, nails, and skin were colored with coloring agents made from _____.
    - a. berries
    - b. bark
    - c. minerals
    - d. All answers are correct.   _____

6. In ancient Egypt, the entire bodies of _____ were shaved every third day.
    - a. women
    - b. priests
    - c. kings
    - d. tradesmen   _____

7. Masai warriors wove their front hair into _____ section(s) of tiny braids and the rest of the hair into a queue down the back.
    - a. one
    - b. two
    - c. three
    - d. four   _____

8. During the lifetime of Moses, barbering was available _____.

    a. to the general   c. only for the rich
        population   d. only for priests
    b. only for the poor

                                          _____

9. Alexander the Great's Macedonians troops lost several battles to the _____ as a result of the warriors' beards.

    a. Egyptians   c. Jews
    b. Persians   d. Romans

                                          _____

10. In Rome, clean-shaven faces were the trend until Hadrian came into power in _____.

    a. 342 BC   c. 117 AD
    b. 117 BC   d. 342 AD

                                          _____

11. Noblemen of ancient Gaul indicated their _____ by wearing their hair long.

    a. family role   c. age
    b. religion   d. rank

                                          _____

12. The _____ abolished the practice of tonsure in 1972.

    a. Greeks   c. Roman Catholic Church
    b. Egyptians   d. State barbering board

                                          _____

13. British barristers wore gray wigs in _____ -century England.

    a. fifteenth   c. seventeenth
    b. sixteenth   d. nineteenth

                                          _____

14. In 3000 BC, _____ were shaving with obsidian blades.

    a. Mesopotamians   c. Romans
    b. Egyptians   d. Greeks

                                          _____

15. During the _____, monks and priests were the physicians.

    a. Renaissance   c. Middle Ages
    b. reign of Alexander   d. nineteenth century
       the Great

                                          _____

16. In _____ AD, the barber-surgeons formed their first organization in France.

    a. 141   c. 1252
    b. 1096   d. 1764

                                          _____

17. The bottom end-cap of modern barber poles represents
    ____.
    a. the basin that was used as a vessel to catch the blood during bloodletting
    b. the colors of the French flag
    c. the shampoo bowl that is used to wash client's hair
    d. None of the answers are correct.   _____

18. The colors of the barber pole represented blood, _____, and bandages.
    a. hair   c. skin
    b. teeth   d. veins   _____

19. During the _____, employer organizations of barbers were known as master barber groups.
    a. late 1800s   c. mid-1900s
    b. early 1900s   d. late 1900s   _____

20. The Terminal Methods system was enacted in _____ in New York City.
    a. 1872   c. 1916
    b. 1896   d. 1925   _____

CHAPTER 3—PROFESSIONAL IMAGE

Multiple Choice

1. The image _____ is a reflection of you as an individual.
   - a. of your position
   - b. of your success
   - c. you project to others
   - d. you see in the mirror

   _____

2. Your _____ is an impression you project to others.
   - a. image
   - b. attire
   - c. personality
   - d. None of the answers are correct.

   _____

3. Your professional image is shaped by _____.
   - a. friends and colleagues
   - b. clothing and hairstyle
   - c. prior learning and life experiences
   - d. None of the answers are correct.

   _____

4. Life skills are the _____ that prepare you for living as a mature adult in a challenging and often complicated world.
   - a. rules
   - b. tools and guidelines
   - c. ethics
   - d. morals

   _____

5. Patience and _____ are life skills.
   - a. intelligence
   - b. adaptability
   - c. beauty
   - d. wealth

   _____

6. Persistence and a "can-do" attitude are important _____.
   - a. goals
   - b. life skills
   - c. types of common sense
   - d. morals

   _____

7. Values consist of _____.
   - a. what we think
   - b. how we fee
   - c. how we act
   - d. All answers are correct.

   _____

8. Beliefs are specific attitudes that occur as a result of our _____ and that have a strong influence on how we act or behave in situations.
   - a. personality
   - b. values
   - c. education
   - d. job

   _____

9. Personality is expressed through _____.
   - a. beliefs
   - b. values
   - c. income
   - d. gestures

   _____

10. There is an old adage that says, "The only difference between _____ is your attitude."
    a. a good day and a bad day
    b. a good hair day and a bad hair day
    c. success and failure
    d. values and morals   _____

11. Being _____ is part of diplomacy.
    a. honest   c. tactful
    b. silent   d. aggressive   _____

12. Sensitivity is a combination of _____.
    a. understanding and honesty
    b. empathy and education
    c. acceptance, honesty, and morality
    d. understanding, empathy, and acceptance   _____

13. An example of courtesy is _____.
    a. being flexible about when you show up to work
    b. making jokes while working
    c. buying lunch for your coworkers every day
    d. being considerate of those with whom you work   _____

14. Personal hygiene involves all of the following except _____.
    a. daily bathing   c. teeth brushing
    b. use of deodorant   d. dry cleaning your clothes   _____

15. The best choice of clothing for working in a barbershop would be _____.
    a. baggy jeans   c. a tuxedo
    b. clean and pressed trousers   d. a sweatsuit   _____

16. During sleep, _____.
    a. the heart rests
    b. the hair stops growing
    c. body tissues and organs are rebuilt
    d. body tissues are broken down   _____

17. Eight hours of sleep _____.
    a. is too little for everyone
    b. is too little for most people
    c. is too much for everyone
    d. may be too much or too little depending on the person   _____

18. Good nutrition includes getting enough _____.
    a. meat
    b. salt
    c. water
    d. juice
    _____

19. Good posture _____.
    a. lessens fatigue
    b. reduces the opportunity for physical problems
    c. helps create an image of confidence
    d. All answers are correct.
    _____

20. Stand with _____ when standing behind the chair.
    a. a straight spine
    b. toes pointing outward
    c. your chin pointing down
    d. stiff shoulders
    _____

21. The _____ should be aligned with the knees when sitting with correct posture.
    a. arms
    b. shoulders
    c. soles of the feet
    d. hips
    _____

22. Due to their profession, barbers are particularly susceptible to problems in their _____.
    a. back
    b. hair
    c. skin
    d. chest
    _____

23. When holding your arms away from your body while working, position your arms _____.
    a. straight
    b. so that your hands point down
    c. against your sides
    d. at less than a 60-degree angle
    _____

24. Clients should be greeted _____.
    a. in a high-pitched tone
    b. reluctantly
    c. by last name
    d. by first name
    _____

25. Avoid talking about _____ in the barbershop.
    a. politics
    b. sports
    c. movies you have seen
    d. the weather
    _____

26. _____ enhances your image.
    a. Listening more than speaking
    b. A critical approach
    c. Tapping your foot
    d. Sharing your personal problems
    _____

27. _____ is an important part of communication.
    a. Image
    b. Grooming
    c. Conversational ability
    d. Moral character
    _____

28. When determining a client's expectations, repeat your interpretation of what the client said _____.
    a. only if asked
    b. before asking any questions
    c. after the client's description
    d. None of the answers are correct.   _____

29. State boards set the _____ that all barbers who work in that state must follow.
    a. ethical standards
    b. tax rules
    c. wage structure
    d. All of the answers are correct.   _____

30. _____ is an example of ethical behavior.
    a. Building your reputation at the expense of others
    b. Making difficult promises
    c. Expecting certain conduct from employees
    d. Selling clients products that they do not want   _____

31. Compartmentalization _____.
    a. can lead to mental illness
    b. helps you to keep your personal and work/school lives separate
    c. is a set of ethical standards set by state barber boards
    d. involves listening and speaking skills   _____

32. Motivation is the ignition for _____.
    a. success
    b. empathy
    c. failure
    d. None of the answers are correct.   _____

33. _____ leads to discovering novel solutions to challenges.
    a. Creativity
    b. Praise
    c. Criticism
    d. Structure   _____

34. A goal with a time frame of a year or less is a _____ goal.
    a. meaningless
    b. short-term
    c. medium-term
    d. long-term   _____

35. Time management includes _____.
    a. taking on all available tasks
    b. prioritizing tasks
    c. ignoring problem-solving techniques
    d. acting on instinct   _____

CHAPTER 4—MICROBIOLOGY

Multiple Choice

1. _____ are a type of microorganism.
   - a. Mammals
   - b. Reptiles
   - c. Protozoa
   - d. Nematodes
   _____

2. Pathogens are microorganisms that are capable of causing infectious diseases in _____.
   - a. only plants
   - b. only animals
   - c. plants or animals
   - d. plants, animals, or microorganisms
   _____

3. Bacteria only have one cell and are called _____ microorganisms.
   - a. microcellular
   - b. unicellular
   - c. single
   - d. None of the answers are correct.
   _____

4. Disease can be produced by _____ bacteria.
   - a. viral
   - b. nonpathogenic
   - c. pathogenic
   - d. probiotic
   _____

5. Staphylococci bacteria cause _____.
   - a. pneumonia
   - b. MRSA
   - c. blood poisoning
   - d. gonorrhea
   _____

6. Diplococci bacteria _____ and cause pneumonia and gonorrhea.
   - a. grow singly
   - b. grow in pairs
   - c. are rod-shaped
   - d. are curved
   _____

7. Cocci bacteria are transmitted by all of the following except _____.
   - a. active motility
   - b. air
   - c. dust
   - d. water
   _____

8. The outer part of a bacterium is the _____.
   - a. cytoplasm
   - b. spore
   - c. cell wall
   - d. bacilli
   _____

9. Microorganisms multiply well in _____ conditions.
   - a. dry
   - b. warm
   - c. cool
   - d. clean
   _____

10. During mitosis, 16,000,000 microbes can be created by one bacterium in a _____ period.
    a. 30-second
    b. 10-minute
    c. 6-hour
    d. 12-hour _____

11. When the body is unable to cope with _____, an infection occurs.
    a. pus
    b. bacteria and their harmful toxins
    c. nonpathogenic bacteria
    d. All of the answers are correct. _____

12. To limit the spread of MRSA, _____.
    a. cover scrapes and cuts
    b. avoid contact with other people's wounds
    c. avoid contact with other people's personal items
    d. All answers are correct. _____

13. A contagious disease _____.
    a. spreads from one person to another by contact
    b. spreads throughout the infected person's bloodstream
    c. attacks a large number of people in one area
    d. is only caused by bacteria _____

14. Open sores, pus, and unclean hands _____.
    a. are all commonly seen in well-run barbershops
    b. will always cause an epidemic
    c. may be a source of contagion
    d. will always cause a general infection _____

15. _____ or an open sore can spread body fluids to a razor during shaving.
    a. Shaving lather
    b. A gloved hand
    c. A hair
    d. A blemish _____

16. The _____ is are one way that pathogenic bacteria or viruses typically enter the body.
    a. mouth
    b. fingernails
    c. scalp
    d. hair _____

17. The body _____ using perspiration.
    a. fights infection
    b. heats up
    c. becomes infected
    d. None of the answers are correct. _____

18. Swelling is an example of a(n) _____ symptom.
    a. subjective
    b. objective
    c. imagined
    d. transient _____

19. Viruses cause _____.
    a. pneumonia   c. gonorrhea
    b. common colds   d. MRSA   _____

20. _____ is a defense against viruses.
    a. Vaccination   c. Fungi
    b. Antibiotics   d. Mitosis   _____

21. Hepatitis B can cause lifelong hepatitis infection,
    cirrhosis of the liver, and _____.
    a. liver failure   c. death
    b. liver cancer   d. All answers are correct. _____

22. Hepatitis B _____.
    a. usually lasts three weeks
    b. is uncommon in the United States
    c. vaccinations are available
    d. causes sepsis   _____

23. Once infected with HIV, a person _____.
    a. will show immediate symptoms
    b. cannot pass on the virus for 11 years
    c. can pass on the virus without having symptoms
    d. will develop AIDS within one year   _____

24. The lymphoreticular system provides storage
    for mature _____.
    a. M cells   c. lymph
    b. blood   d. lymphocytes   _____

25. A retrovirus such as _____ uses the reproductive
    processes of the host cell to duplicate itself.
    a. HIV   c. hepatitis C
    b. smallpox   d. Cocci   _____

26. HIV is difficult to destroy once it locks into T cells in the
    _____.
    a. lungs   c. liver
    b. brain   d. bloodstream   _____

27. ARC is _____ of HIV.
    a. stage 1   c. stage 3
    b. stage 2   d. the final stage   _____

28. Before and after servicing each client, barbers
    should _____.
    a. change their clothes
    b. wash their hands with an antibacterial soap
    c. use a gel hand sanitizer
    d. None of the answers are correct.   _____

29. If you cut, nick, or scrape yourself, _____.
    a. treat the wound immediately and cover it
    b. go home and take the rest of the day off
    c. call 911
    d. you must proceed to the hospital as recommended
       by the state barber board   _____

30. The fungi classification includes all of the following
    except _____.
    a. algae   c. rust
    b. mold   d. yeast   _____

31. _____ and pesticides should be used to decontaminate
    tools that have come into contact with scabies.
    a. Fungicides   c. Ultraviolet light
    b. Steam   d. Disinfectants   _____

32. Natural immunity is the natural resistance to disease
    that is _____.
    a. wholly inherited
    b. wholly developed through hygienic living
    c. partially inherited and partially developed
       through hygienic living
    d. acquired through vaccination   _____

33. Acquired immunity comes from _____.
    a. your parents   c. antibiotics
    b. hygienic living   d. overcoming disease   _____

34. A human disease carrier _____.
    a. is immune to a disease but can infect others
    b. is not immune to a disease and can infect others
    c. is immune to a disease and cannot infect others
    d. is not immune to a disease and cannot
       infect others   _____

35. Stage 3 HIV infection is _____.
    a. ARC   c. hepatitis A
    b. full blown AIDS   d. MRSA   _____

36. _____ attaches itself to special molecules on T cells.
    a. HIV   c. Hepatitis
    b. The B cell   d. Scabies   _____

CHAPTER 5—INFECTION CONTROL AND SAFE WORK PRACTICES

Multiple Choice

1. The spread of contagious diseases is minimized by _____.
   - a. close contact with other people
   - b. frequent visits to the doctor
   - c. the implementation of infection control measures
   - d. All of the answers are correct.   _____

2. _____ are not responsible for regulating the practice of barbering.
   - a. Local agencies
   - b. Barbershop owners
   - c. State agencies
   - d. Federal agencies   _____

3. The EPA is responsible for developing and enforcing the regulations of environmental laws in an effort to _____.
   - a. protect local businesses
   - b. avoid lawsuits
   - c. minimize human interaction with the environment
   - d. protect human health and the environment   _____

4. The FDA enforces rules and regulations associated with _____ purchased and used by the public.
   - a. foods
   - b. drugs
   - c. cosmetics
   - d. All answers are correct.   _____

5. _____ is/are one of the cosmetic preparations typically used in the barbershop.
   - a. Razors
   - b. Clippers
   - c. Hair spray
   - d. Toothpaste   _____

6. _____ products are not required to display a list of ingredients on the label.
   - a. Professional
   - b. Retail
   - c. Over-the-counter
   - d. None of the answers are correct.   _____

7. _____ was passed in 1970 to assure, regulate, and enforce safe and healthful working conditions in the workplace.
   - a. FDA
   - b. OSHA
   - c. MSDS
   - d. EPA   _____

8. The Bloodborne Pathogens Standard helps to protect
   _____ from being at risk from cross-infection.
      a. the public   c. barbershop clients
      b. employees   d. All of the answers
                                 are correct.   _____

9. The Hazard Communication Rule includes requirements
   for _____.
      a. pharmacists and technicians
      b. all importers
      c. anyone who uses drugs
      d. chemical manufacturers and importers   _____

10. MSDSs are available from _____.
       a. a barber school   c. the product manufacturer
       b. the FDA   d. the EPA   _____

11. Labeling refers to the listing of ingredients and the
    appropriate _____ on the packaging of a product.
       a. hazard warning   c. uses
       b. price   d. administration   _____

12. According to the Right-to-Know law, one of the _____'s
    responsibilities is to maintain Material Safety Data
    Sheets and have them available upon request.
       a. government   c. employer
       b. employee   d. client   _____

13. _____' health, safety, and welfare while receiving
    services in the barbershop is protected by state
    regulatory agencies.
       a. Employers   c. Employees
       b. Consumers   d. All answers are correct.   _____

14. The key to effective infection control is _____, which is
    primarily the responsibility of barbershop personnel.
       a. the prevention of the transmission of microorganisms
       b. periodic cleaning
       c. keeping all germs outside of the barbershop
       d. treating illness   _____

15. Decontamination is _____.
       a. the prevention of the spread of disease
       b. the destruction of pathogens within the body
       c. the removal of pathogens and other substances
          from tools or surfaces
       d. a method for treating disease   _____

16. The _____ level of decontamination is sanitation or cleaning.
    a. lowest
    b. second
    c. fourth
    d. highest
    _____

17. Sanitation or cleaning involves _____.
    a. washing with water only
    b. washing with soaps or detergents
    c. chemicals such as hydrogen peroxide
    d. chemicals such as bleach
    _____

18. Sterilization is the _____ level of effective decontamination.
    a. lowest
    b. second
    c. fourth
    d. highest
    _____

19. _____ used to destroy harmful microorganisms are called disinfectants.
    a. Cleaning implements
    b. Light rays
    c. Soaps
    d. Prepared chemical substances
    _____

20. Sanitation or cleaning includes _____.
    a. bleaching
    b. hand washing
    c. immersion in hospital-grade disinfectant
    d. None of the answers are correct
    _____

21. Public sanitation is the application of measures to _____.
    a. promote less contact between people
    b. eradicate infectious diseases
    c. develop new medicines
    d. promote public health and prevent the spread of infectious diseases
    _____

22. Chemical or _____ agents are used to decontaminate barbering tools and shop surfaces.
    a. engineered
    b. natural
    c. biological
    d. physical
    _____

23. An example of a physical decontamination agent is _____.
    a. steam
    b. antiseptics
    c. disinfectants
    d. phenol
    _____

24. The electric UV sanitizer is a(n) _____ disinfection
method commonly used in modern barbershops.
    a. antiseptic   c. septic
    b. physical   d. chemical   _____

25. Substances that may kill, retard, or prevent the growth
of bacteria and _____ are antiseptics.
    a. can generally be used safely on the skin
    b. should never be used on the skin
    c. can be used only on the hair
    d. are generally used only in hospitals   _____

26. The chemical agents used to destroy _____ are
disinfectants.
    a. most viruses and some bacteria
    b. most bacteria and some viruses
    c. all viruses but not bacteria
    d. all bacteria but not viruses   _____

27. In crystal form, _____ is used as an antiseptic.
    a. isopropyl alcohol   c. ethyl alcohol
    b. boric acid   d. sodium hydrochlorite   _____

28. Immersing implements with sharp cutting edges in
bleach for a minimum of 10 minutes serves to _____
them.
    a. disinfect   c. grade
    b. clean   d. destroy   _____

29. The EPA is responsible for _____.
    a. testing disinfectants
    b. approving all disinfectants
    c. approving new-to-the-market disinfectants
    d. making claims about the effectiveness
       of disinfectants   _____

30. Products that will kill either the staphylococcus or
salmonella organisms, but not both, have a _____ level
of disinfection efficacy.
    a. limited   c. hospital-grade
    b. general   d. hospital-grade
                                     tuberculocidal   _____

31. Hospital-grade tuberculocidal is the _____ level of
disinfection.
    a. highest   c. third
    b. second   d. lowest   _____

32. Most _____ solutions disinfect implements in
    10–15 minutes.
    a. quat   c. limited disinfection
    b. phenol   d. general disinfection   _____

33. Rubber and plastic materials should be used with care
    because they may become softened or discolored with
    continued _____ use.
    a. phenol   c. alcohol
    b. quat   d. bleach   _____

34. _____ disinfectants include pine oil.
    a. Petroleum distillate   c. Phenol
    b. Sodium hypochlorite   d. Quat   _____

35. A 50 to 60 percent _____ alcohol solution may be used
    on the skin as an antiseptic.
    a. pine   c. isopropyl
    b. phenol   d. ethyl   _____

36. H-42 Disinfectant and _____ are multipurpose
    formulations that can be used on surfaces and
    implements.
    a. Barbicide®   c. Lysol®
    b. Pine-Sol®   d. Clippercide®   _____

37. The four functions that commercial prepared products
    perform are cleaning, _____, lubrication, and/or cooling.
    a. satiation   c. heating
    b. disinfection   d. None of the answers
                                  are correct.   _____

38. Dilute _____ with water to achieve the required
    strength.
    a. concentrates   c. Lysol®
    b. petroleum distillates   d. blade wash   _____

39. A solute is _____.
    a. a type of disinfectant
    b. the substance in which something is dissolved
    c. the substance that is dissolved
    d. a concentrated solution   _____

40. The percentage of solute is indicated by the _____ of the
    solution.
    a. price   c. strength
    b. concentration   d. purity   _____

41. _____ cabinets used to store disinfected tools and implements are called ultraviolet-ray sanitizers.
    a. Glass   c. Wood
    b. Plastic   d. Metal   _____

42. A cabinet sanitizer is an airtight cabinet containing an active fumigant such as _____.
    a. formalin   c. steam
    b. quats   d. phenols   _____

43. After using a wet sanitizer for the recommended amount of time and rinsing the implements, _____.
    a. dry them with a clean towel
    b. place in a dry cabinet
    c. wash again with soap and water
    d. use the implements immediately   _____

44. To disinfect clippers, pour blade wash into a _____ container.
    a. glass   c. disposable
    b. plastic   d. All answers are correct.   _____

45. Work surfaces should be disinfected with an EPA-registered, hospital-grade tuberculocidal disinfectant _____.
    a. once a month   c. twice a day
    b. once a day   d. before and after
                              each client   _____

46. Standard precautions cover bodily fluids and body sites and were developed by the _____.
    a. CDC   c. FDA
    b. EPA   d. state barber boards   _____

47. Blood-spill disinfection is required when _____.
    a. a client sustains a cut during a service
    b. a client has a bloody nose before a service procedure and leaves the shop
    c. a client exhibits signs of infection
    d. None of the answers are correct   _____

48. When chemical solution becomes _____, change it.
    a. dirty   c. contaminated
    b. cloudy   d. All answers are correct.   _____

49. 70 degrees Fahrenheit is _____ for a barbershop.
    a. too warm   c. an ideal temperature
    b. too cold   d. inappropriate   _____

50. When implements are used, they should be _____.
    a. immediately cleaned and disinfected
    b. put aside until the end of the day
    c. washed with soap and used again
    d. immediately used again   _____

51. If a client is cut during a service procedure, _____.
    a. the client should be informed
    b. the barber should not tell anyone
    c. the barber will be fired
    d. the barber's license will be suspended   _____

CHAPTER 6—IMPLEMENTS, TOOLS, AND EQUIPMENT

Multiple Choice

1. Well-tempered metal implements and electric tools will provide years of dependable service _____.
   a. when used infrequently
   b. when polished daily
   c. when taken care of properly
   d. None of the answers are correct.
   _____

2. Depending on the type of service, _____.
   a. a bone comb is normally preferred
   b. the comb selection may vary
   c. let the client decide which comb he prefers
   d. select the cheapest comb
   _____

3. Wide-toothed combs are preferred for _____.
   a. general-purpose use
   b. flat-top styles
   c. trimming mustaches and areas around the ears
   d. detangling or chemical processing
   _____

4. Use a taper comb for _____.
   a. chemically processing hair
   b. those areas where a gradual blending of the hair is required
   c. general-purpose combing
   d. creating a flap-top style
   _____

5. Use a pick comb for _____.
   a. mustache trims
   b. spreading relaxer creams
   c. combing straight hair
   d. combing through tight curl patterns
   _____

6. When should combs be disinfected?
   a. When they are brand new
   b. At the beginning of the day
   c. Before serving each client
   d. At the end of the day
   _____

7. Use a black comb when cutting _____ hair.
   a. permed
   b. straight
   c. dark-colored
   d. blonde
   _____

8. _____ is not commonly used for brush bristles.
   a. Plastic
   b. Nylon
   c. Metal
   d. Boar hair
   _____

9. French style shears _____.
    a. contain a brace for the thumb
    b. are almost never used in barbershops
    c. contain a brace for the little finger
    d. do not have a brace for the little finger   _____

10. The main parts of the shears do not include the _____.
    a. points   c. tang
    b. cutting edges   d. grind   _____

11. A shear measuring 7 inches using the German method
    will be _____ inches using the Japanese method.
    a. 4   c. 6.5
    b. 6   d. 7.5   _____

12. The inside construction of the blade and the _____ is
    called the grind.
    a. way it is cut in preparation for sharpening
       and polishing
    b. size and shape of the finger grip
    c. way that the shear blade is measured
    d. sharpness of the blade   _____

13. When there is a(n) _____ on the cutting surface of the
    blade, this is a beveled edge.
    a. clamshell shape   c. half-moon shape
    b. angle   d. straight edge   _____

14. The outside of a convex blade edge has a(n) _____.
    a. clamshell or   c. combination of angles
       half-moon shape   and planes
    b. angular shape   d. serrated edge   _____

15. Thinning shears are also called _____ shears.
    a. bending   c. razor
    b. hybrid   d. convex   _____

16. The ring finger is inserted into the finger grip of the
    still blade and the little finger _____.
    a. rests on the finger brace
    b. rests on the moving edge
    c. wraps under the shears
    d. does not touch the shears   _____

17. Transfer the comb to the opposite hand and palm it
    ___.
    a. when blow-drying the hair
    b. after cutting a section of hair
    c. before combing the section of hair into position
       for cutting
    d. after combing the section of hair into position
       for cutting _____

18. To check the tension of the shears, hold the shears _____.
    a. horizontally by the thumb grip
    b. vertically by the thumb grip
    c. horizontally by the still blade
    d. vertically by the still blade _____

19. Wiping hair from under the tension screw is the _____
    step in cleaning shears.
    a. first   c. third
    b. second   d. last _____

20. Trimmers are essential for _____.
    a. finish and detail work c. longer hairstyles
    b. short haircuts   d. mustache work _____

21. The visible parts of an electric clipper are the _____,
    still blade, heel, switch, set or power screw, and
    conducting cord.
    a. blade cover   c. shear
    b. finger grip   d. cutting blade _____

22. Compared to magnetic clippers, pivot motor clippers
    produce _____ the number of blade strokes.
    a. twice   c. four times
    b. three times   d. five times _____

23. A trimmer is another name for a(n) _____.
    a. razor   c. shear
    b. outliner   d. clipper _____

24. Carbon steel is used to make _____.
    a. combs   c. clipper blades
    b. brush handles   d. brush bristles _____

25. The 0000 blade _____.
    a. produces the   c. is never used for cutting
       closest cut   hair
    b. is the largest size d. None of the answers
                            are correct. _____

26. Clipper guards _____.
    a. cut the hair shorter
    b. allow the hair to be left longer
    c. are always used in barbershops
    d. protect the client's scalp

    _____

27. To cut the hair 1⅛" to 1⅜" long, use _____ clipper blades.
    a. ½"   c. 1.25"
    b. 1"   d. 1.4"

    _____

28. It is recommended that blades be _____ before, during (as needed), and after each use.
    a. wiped   c. washed
    b. sanitized   d. oiled

    _____

29. Keep the grease chamber should be kept about two-thirds full when using _____ clippers.
    a. cutting blade   c. magnetic
    b. pivot motor   d. rotary motor

    _____

30. Razors are used for _____.
    a. facial shaves   c. behind-the-ear areas
    b. neck shaves   d. All answers are correct.

    _____

31. Honing and stropping _____ the conventional straight razor.
    a. maintain the cutting c. disinfect
       edge on   d. are not required for
    b. clean

    _____

32. The changeable-blade straight razor _____.
    a. is the least popular for barbering
    b. is the most popular for barbering
    c. must be honed and stropped
    d. does not give a close shave

    _____

33. Razor balance refers to the _____.
    a. polish of the blade's surface
    b. shape of the blade
    c. degree of hardness of the blade
    d. weight and length of the blade relative to that of the handle

    _____

34. Razor grind refers to the _____.
    a. polish of the blade's surface
    b. shape of the blade
    c. degree of hardness of the blade
    d. weight and length of the blade relative to
       that of the handle   _____

35. The style of a razor indicates _____.
    a. where it was made   c. the materials that make
    b. its shape and   up the razor
       design   d. the grind   _____

36. After use, a razor should be cleaned and _____, and
    a little oil applied to the cutting edge.
    a. ground   c. stropped
    b. honed   d. disinfected   _____

37. A _____ hone is gray or brown in color.
    a. water   c. Belgian
    b. clay   d. Swaty   _____

38. The Belgian hone is a natural hone _____.
    a. that should not be used with lather
    b. cut from rock formations
    c. that is quick cutting
    d. made of carborundum   _____

39. Combination hones _____.
    a. are never used in professional barbershops
    b. are made of rock
    c. are used by most barbers
    d. are manufactured in Belgium   _____

40. The _____ strop is made of linen.
    a. canvas   c. German
    b. French   d. Belgian   _____

41. A Russian strop _____.
    a. does not require   c. is made of linen
       breaking in   d. is considered one
    b. is made in Russia   of the best   _____

42. _____ cleans the leather strop, preserves its finish,
    and also improves its draw and sharpening qualities.
    a. Disinfectant   c. A Russian strop
    b. Strop dressing   d. A water hone   _____

43. The _____ position when honing a razor involves placing the razor on the upper far left corner of the hone on its back.
    a. first   c. third
    b. second   d. last   _____

44. Draw the razor backward in a diagonal line across the hone to _____.
    a. break in the hone   c. correct an over-honed edge
    b. finish honing a razor   d. achieve over-honing   _____

45. Attach the strop to the arm of the barber chair _____.
    a. to stretch it, then hold with the left hand
    b. if the barber has a weak grip
    c. before honing the razor
    d. when stropping the razor   _____

46. Lather receptacles _____.
    a. are containers used to hold or dispense lather for shaving
    b. should only be used if no lather mug is available
    c. are not recommended by state barbering boards
    d. None of the answers are correct.   _____

47. The number 3 size of lather brush _____.
    a. is too large
    b. is favored by most barbers
    c. is only used for very thick beards
    d. is only used for very curly beards   _____

48. Freestyle drying can be performed by moving the dryer back and forth sideways, _____.
    a. allowing the hair to fall naturally into place
    b. to create a stylized effect
    c. to avoid drying the hair too quickly
    d. and then up and down   _____

49. The main function of the galvanic machine is to introduce _____ products into the skin during a facial.
    a. disinfecting   c. acidic
    b. alkaline   d. water-soluble   _____

50. The comedone extractor is a metallic implement with a screwed attachment at each end used to _____.
    a. press out whiteheads   c. introduce galvanic current
    b. press out blackheads   d. None of the answers
                                       are correct.   _____

CHAPTER 7—ANATOMY AND PHYSIOLOGY

Multiple Choice

1. Anatomy is the study of the _____.
   a. shape and structure of an organism's body and the relationship of one body part to another
   b. mechanical, physical, and biochemical functions and activities of each body part
   c. growth of all life forms
   d. anatomical structures of an organism that are easily observable through visible inspection   _____

2. _____ used in the practice of barbering might affect physiological activities of the body.
   a. Massage manipulations
   b. Heat
   c. Absorptive products
   d. All answers are correct.   _____

3. Barbers are particularly concerned with the histology of the skin and the _____.
   a. hair
   b. nails
   c. sweat glands
   d. All answers are correct.   _____

4. Cells are the _____.
   a. atomic and indivisible unit that makes up human life
   b. sole subject when studying anatomy
   c. smallest visible particle
   d. basic units of structure and function of all living things   _____

5. The nucleus is _____.
   a. the most important organelle within the cell
   b. the outside of the cell
   c. filled with protoplasm
   d. the place where cells store food   _____

6. Protoplasm is found _____.
   a. only outside the nucleus
   b. only inside the nucleus
   c. in the nucleus and cytoplasm
   d. in the nucleus, cytoplasm, and cell membrane   _____

7. During mitosis, cells divide into _____ daughter cell(s).
   a. one
   b. two
   c. three
   d. four   _____

8. Anabolism is the _____ that builds up cellular tissues.
   a. constructive metabolism
   b. protoplasm
   c. mitosis
   d. organelle _____

9. During catabolism, the cells _____ in order to release the energy needed to perform specialized functions.
   a. absorb food and water
   b. consume what they have absorbed
   c. divide
   d. reproduce _____

10. Which of the following is not one of the five main types of tissue?
    a. Muscular
    b. Liquid
    c. Nerve
    d. Catabolic _____

11. Liquid tissue carries _____ through the body.
    a. cytoplasm
    b. protoplasm
    c. food and waste products
    d. messages _____

12. Muscular tissue _____.
    a. supports, protects, and binds together other tissues
    b. provides a protective covering
    c. contracts and moves various parts of the body
    d. carries messages from the brain _____

13. Epithelial tissue _____.
    a. carries hormones through the body
    b. includes bone and fat
    c. controls body functions
    d. is a protective covering on body surfaces _____

14. The kidneys _____.
    a. control body movements
    b. excrete water and other waste products
    c. digest food
    d. remove toxic products of digestion _____

15. Systems are groups of _____ that act together to perform one or more functions within the body.
    a. organs
    b. tissues
    c. nerves
    d. cells _____

16. The excretory system _____.
    a. includes the heart and blood vessels
    b. purifies the body by the elimination of waste matter
    c. affects the growth and health of the entire body
    d. enables breathing   _____

17. The circulatory system consists of the _____.
    a. heart and blood vessels
    b. mouth and intestines
    c. brain, spinal cord, and nerves
    d. lungs   _____

18. The endocrine system _____.
    a. controls the circulation of blood
    b. includes the kidneys
    c. consists of specialized glands
    d. is responsible for eliminating carbon dioxide   _____

19. Bone is composed of one-third _____ and two-thirds
    minerals.
    a. water   c. oxygen
    b. animal matter   d. nerves   _____

20. The pelvis _____.
    a. is an immovable joint   c. consists of only one bone
    b. is a movable joint   d. is one of the cranial bones _____

21. The occipital bone _____.
    a. joins all the cranial bones together
    b. is located between the eye sockets
    c. forms the top of the cranium
    d. is the hindmost bone of the skull   _____

22. The ethmoid bone _____.
    a. forms the bridge of the nose
    b. is the light, spongy bone between the eye sockets
    c. forms the sides of the head
    d. is a fragile bone forming the cheeks   _____

23. Which of the following facial bones is a single bone as
    opposed to a pair?
    a. maxillary   c. palatine
    b. vomer   d. lacrimal   _____

24. The two zygomatic bones _____.
    a. form the prominence of the cheeks
    b. forms the upper jaw
    c. are located in the front part of the eye
    d. are located in the throat   _____

25. The two maxillary bones _____.
    a. are also called malar bones
    b. join to form the whole upper jaw
    c. form the bridge of the nose
    d. are the largest and strongest in the face   _____

26. *Thorax* is a term for the _____.
    a. throat   c. thumb
    b. forearm   d. chest   _____

27. The humerus is located in the _____.
    a. arm   c. leg
    b. skull   d. chest   _____

28. The ulna is the inner and larger bone of the _____.
    a. hand   c. leg
    b. forearm   d. chest   _____

29. Each _____ contains three phalanges.
    a. arm   c. leg
    b. finger   d. foot   _____

30. Myology is the study of _____.
    a. bones   c. the entire body
    b. muscles   d. the systems of the body   _____

31. The muscular system relies upon the _____ systems for
    its activities and proper operation.
    a. skeletal and nervous   c. skeletal and digestive
    b. excretory and nervous d. nervous and circulatory _____

32. Striated muscles _____.
    a. are controlled by will
    b. make up the heart
    c. are found in internal organs
    d. are not found in the face   _____

33. Non-striated muscles are found in the _____.
    a. stomach   c. arm
    b. leg   d. face   _____

34. The insertion of a muscle refers to _____.
    a. its center
    b. the more movable attachment
    c. the more fixed attachment
    d. the cells that make up the muscle   _____

35. Skeletal muscles _____.
    a. are located inside bones
    b. are also called cardiac muscles
    c. are attached to bones
    d. are attached to the skin   _____

36. The belly of a muscle is the _____.
    a. outside of the muscle   c. moving end
    b. attached end   d. center   _____

37. _____ stimulate(s) muscular tissue.
    a. Cold pressure   c. Chemicals
    b. Visible light   d. Bacteria   _____

38. The epicranius _____.
    a. is a tendon   c. draws the scalp forward
    b. draws the scalp   d. covers the top of
       backward   the skull   _____

39. The corrugator is a muscle of the _____.
    a. nose   c. eyebrow
    b. scalp   d. eye socket   _____

40. The procerus is a muscle of the _____.
    a. cheek   c. eye
    b. tongue   d. nose   _____

41. The buccinator _____.
    a. draws the corner of the mouth back
    b. compresses the cheeks and expels air between the lips
    c. wrinkles the lips
    d. depresses the lower lip   _____

42. The mentalis causes _____.
    a. wrinkling in the chin
    b. compressed cheeks
    c. puckered lips
    d. wrinkles across the bridge of the nose   _____

43. The auricularis posterior _____ .
    a. draws down the corner of the mouth
    b. is located above the ear
    c. draws the ear backward
    d. draws the ear upward   _____

44. The platysma is a broad muscle extending from the chest
    and shoulder muscles to the side of the _____ .
    a. neck   c. chin
    b. waist   d. arm   _____

45. The adductor muscles are part of the _____ .
    a. hand   c. leg
    b. foot   d. arm   _____

46. The nervous system _____ .
    a. is the smallest system, containing only the brain
    b. is one of the least important systems of the body
    c. controls and coordinates the functions of all the
       other systems
    d. None of the answers are correct.   _____

47. The nervous system has three main subdivisions: _____ .
    a. peripheral, central, and cranial
    b. cerebrospinal, peripheral, and autonomic
    c. cranial, autonomic, and sensory
    d. sensory, motor, and mixed   _____

48. The cerebrospinal nervous system includes the _____ .
    a. spinal nerves   c. spinal cord
    b. brain   d. All answers are correct.   _____

49. The peripheral nervous system is made up of _____ nerve
    fibers.
    a. anabolic   c. sensory and motor
    b. temporal and frontal   d. connective   _____

50. The brain _____ .
    a. controls sensation, muscles, and glandular activity
    b. carries messages through the body
    c. is part of the autonomic nervous system
    d. consciously regulates breathing   _____

51. Thirty-one pairs of spinal nerves _____.
    a. are distributed to the muscles and skin of the trunk and limbs
    b. control all mental activities
    c. function independently of human will
    d. weigh 44 to 48 ounces   _____

52. Axons _____.
    a. carry impulses away from the cell body to the muscles and organs
    b. carry impulses to the cell body
    c. are located outside of the brain only
    d. are located only in the spinal cord   _____

53. Nerves are long, white cords made up of _____.
    a. autonomic muscle   c. single nerve fibers
    b. brain tissue   d. bundles of nerve fibers   _____

54. Cranial nerves contain _____ fibers.
    a. connective   c. motor and sensory
    b. parietal and   d. None of the answers
       temporal   are correct.   _____

55. The supratrochlear nerve affects the _____.
    a. external ear
    b. lower eyelids
    c. skin between the eyes and upper sides of the nose
    d. skin of the scalp   _____

56. The auriculotemporal nerve affects the _____.
    a. external ear   c. skin between the eyes
    b. lower eyelid   d. skin of the forehead   _____

57. The greater auricular cervical nerve affects the _____.
    a. scalp
    b. scalp and base of the skull
    c. external ears and the areas in front and back of the ears
    d. front and sides of the neck   _____

58. A resting heartbeat of 72 to 80 beats a minute _____.
    a. indicates a slow pulse
    b. indicates a too rapid pulse
    c. is normal for an adult
    d. is normal for a child   _____

59. Veins carry _____.
    a. deoxygenated blood back to the heart
    b. wastes out of cells
    c. pure blood from the heart
    d. lymph fluid   _____

60. White blood cells _____.
    a. carry oxygen to cells
    b. protect the body from disease
    c. carry waste from cells
    d. None of the answers are correct.   _____

61. The angular artery supplies the _____.
    a. lower lip   c. chin
    b. side of the nose   d. teeth   _____

62. The _____ artery is an important branch of the
    superficial temporal artery.
    a. occipital   c. frontal
    b. auricular   d. angular   _____

63. The skin _____.
    a. eliminates   c. is responsible for
       perspiration   eliminating oils
    b. makes hormones   d. aids in digestion   _____

64. Abdominal breathing involves the _____.
    a. ribs and diaphragm   c. diaphragm and intestines
    b. instestines and lungs d. stomach and ribs   _____

CHAPTER 8—CHEMISTRY

Multiple Choice

1. In the barbershop, chemicals are used for _____.
    a. permanent hair change
    b. disinfection
    c. cleaning
    d. All answers are correct.
    _____

2. Gasoline, synthetic fiber, and plastic are all _____ substances.
    a. organic
    b. inorganic
    c. chemicals
    d. None of the answers are correct.
    _____

3. An example of matter in a solid state is _____.
    a. water
    b. ice
    c. air
    d. steam
    _____

4. Energy is _____.
    a. organic
    b. inorganic
    c. not used in the barbershop
    d. not matter
    _____

5. There are 117 known elements, _____ of which occur naturally on Earth.
    a. 86
    b. 94
    c. 101
    d. 103
    _____

6. Atoms consist of _____.
    a. protons
    b. neutrons
    c. electrons
    d. All answers are correct.
    _____

7. Elemental molecules are chemical combinations of two or more atoms _____.
    a. of the same element
    c. in different states
    b. of different elements
    d. one of which is organic
    _____

8. Burning wood is an example of _____.
    a. pure matter
    b. energy
    c. a physical change
    d. a chemical change
    _____

9. The density of a substance refers to its _____.
    a. amount of water
    b. mass times volume
    c. weight divided by its volume
    d. volume divided by its weight
    _____

10. Ice melting is an example of _____.
    a. a physical change
    b. a chemical change
    c. matter changing to energy
    d. energy changing to matter   _____

11. Which of the following statements does not apply to
    physical mixtures?
    a. They do not involve chemical reactions.
    b. Water is an example.
    c. Solution of hydrogen peroxide is an example.
    d. They are mixed in any proportion.   _____

12. Oxides are compounds of any element combined
    with _____.
    a. hydrogen peroxide   c. acid
    b. salt   d. oxygen   _____

13. Bases are compounds of hydrogen, _____, and oxygen.
    a. a metal   c. carbon
    b. a salt   d. an acid   _____

14. The most abundant chemical is _____.
    a. organic   c. water
    b. carbon   d. oxygen   _____

15. To _____, boil water.
    a. create a chemical   c. create an acid
       change   d. create a salt
    b. destroy microbes   _____

16. A soap solution can be used to determine the _____
    water.
    a. hardness of
    b. chemical properties of
    c. temperature of
    d. number of microbes in   _____

17. Soft water _____.
    a. does not allow soap to lather well
    b. is the best choice for use in a barbershop
    c. should be boiled
    d. should be filtered   _____

18. Hard water contains mineral substances that _____ soap.
    a. harden   c. curdle or precipitate
    b. lather   d. None of the answers
                               are correct.   _____

19. The letters *pH* denote potential hydrogen, the relative degree of _____ of a substance.
    a. acidity or alkalinity   c. ionization
    b. hardness   d. solubility   _____

20. Ionization is the separation of a substance into _____.
    a. salts and water
    b. acids and bases
    c. ions that have opposite electrical charges
    d. ions with the same electrical charges   _____

21. An anion is a _____.
    a. negatively charged ion
    b. positively charged ion
    c. neutral ion
    d. collection of five or more ions   _____

22. When _____ molecules ionize, the hydrogen ion is acidic and the hydroxide ion is alkaline.
    a. carbon   c. nitrogen
    b. water   d. hydroxyl   _____

23. The pH values are arranged on a scale ranging from _____ to 14.
    a. negative 14   c. 1
    b. 0   d. 10   _____

24. A pH of 8 is 10 times more alkaline than a pH of _____.
    a. 4   c. 6
    b. 5   d. 7   _____

25. The pH range of _____ is an average of 5 on the pH scale.
    a. hair and skin   c. air
    b. water   d. alkalis   _____

26. Another term for a base is _____.
    a. acid   c. anion
    b. alkali   d. cation   _____

27. Acid-balanced shampoos and normalizing lotions associated with hydroxide hair relaxers work create an acid-alkali _____ reaction.
    a. reduction   c. oxidation
    b. ion   d. neutralization   _____

28. Slow oxidation occurs in _____.
    a. oxidation haircolors
    b. permanent wave neutralizers
    c. combustion reactions
    d. oxidation haircolors and permanent
       wave neutralizers

    _____

29. In a(n) _____ reaction, the oxidizer is always reduced and
    the reducing agent is always oxidized.
    a. thioglycolate   c. redox
    b. pH   d. neutral

    _____

30. Powders consist of a uniform mixture of _____ that have
    been properly blended, perfumed, and/or tinted.
    a. insoluble substances   c. suspensions
    b. solutions   d. emulsions

    _____

31. Suspensions are uniform mixtures of _____ substances.
    a. two or more   c. chemically related
    b. three or more   d. neutral

    _____

32. A solvent is usually a _____ and dissolves the solute to
    form a solution.
    a. liquid   c. solid
    b. gas   d. powder

    _____

33. Water is _____.
    a. never used as a solvent
    b. a universal solvent
    c. not capable of dissolving other substances
    d. None of the answers is correct.

    _____

34. Solutions containing volatile substances such as _____
    should be stored in a cool place.
    a. water   c. ammonia and alcohol
    b. carbon   d. All of the answers
                                 are correct.

    _____

35. A saturated solution _____.
    a. contains only one substance
    b. can continue to dissolve more solute
    c. indicates that the solution is overmixed
    d. will not dissolve or take up more solute than
       it already holds

    _____

36. An emulsion is a suspension of _____.
    - a. a solid in a gas
    - b. a solid in a liquid
    - c. one liquid in another
    - d. a liquid in a gas   _____

37. A surfactant molecule has two distinct parts: the head of the molecule is _____ and the tail is lipophilic.
    - a. hydrophilic
    - b. hydrophobic
    - c. saturated
    - d. emulsified   _____

38. Medicated soaps are designed to _____.
    - a. help protect against getting dirty
    - b. treat skin problems such as rashes, pimples, and acne
    - c. provide odor-fighting properties
    - d. moisturize the skin   _____

39. To harden the cuticle of the hair shaft, use a(n) _____.
    - a. medicated shampoo
    - b. moisturizing shampoo
    - c. alkaline solution
    - d. acidic solution   _____

40. Liquid cream shampoos are usually fairly thick liquids that contain _____.
    - a. eggs
    - b. medications for special conditions
    - c. either soap or soap jelly
    - d. moisturizing agents   _____

41. Clarifying shampoos should be used _____.
    - a. only when buildup is evident
    - b. to prevent buildup from forming
    - c. every day
    - d. after swimming in chlorine   _____

42. _____ are special chemical agents that are applied to hair to deposit protein or moisture, restore hair strength and body, or protect against possible damage.
    - a. Conditioners
    - b. Shampoos
    - c. Moisturizers
    - d. Rinses   _____

43. Synthetic polymer conditioners are _____.
    - a. used to treat the scalp
    - b. also known as hair masks
    - c. intended for all hair types
    - d. special formulations for use on badly damaged hair   _____

44. Oil mixture tonics contain considerable amounts of alcohol with a(n) _____.
    a. soap jelly
    b. neutralizing agent
    c. oil base
    d. small portion of oil floating on the top _____

45. Styling aids include _____.
    a. shampoos
    b. gels and mousses
    c. conditioners
    d. rinses _____

46. Alum is an aluminum potassium or ammonium sulphate supplied in the form of _____.
    a. a milky liquid
    b. an odorless gas
    c. a clear liquid
    d. crystals or powder _____

47. Glycerin is a(n) _____ substance formed by the decomposition of oils, fats, or fatty acids.
    a. sweet
    b. colorless
    c. odorless
    d. All answers are correct. _____

48. Sodium carbonate _____.
    a. is found in fresh water
    b. is a skin lubricant
    c. removes hair spray
    d. absorbs water from the air _____

CHAPTER 9—ELECTRICITY AND LIGHT THERAPY

Multiple Choice

1. The directional flow of electrons between _____ creates a form of energy called electricity.
   - a. ions
   - b. atoms
   - c. neutrons
   - d. matter _____

2. The flow of electricity along a(n) _____ is an electric current.
   - a. conductor
   - b. insulator
   - c. atom
   - d. element _____

3. Good conductors include watery solutions of acids and _____.
   - a. atoms
   - b. salts
   - c. wires
   - d. bases _____

4. An example of a good insulator is _____.
   - a. metal
   - b. the human body
   - c. cement
   - d. carbon _____

5. The path of electric current from the generating source through conductors and _____ is a complete circuit.
   - a. then through an insulator
   - b. over a long distance
   - c. back to its original source
   - d. None of the answers are correct. _____

6. Direct current is used by _____.
   - a. battery-operated instruments
   - b. rectifiers
   - c. electric clippers
   - d. hair dryers _____

7. Alternating current is used by _____.
   - a. flashlights
   - b. electric clippers
   - c. cellular phones
   - d. converters _____

8. A rectifier might be used by _____.
   - a. a flashlight
   - b. electric clippers
   - c. rechargeable cordless clippers
   - d. hair dryers _____

9. A weak current indicates low _____.
   - a. voltage
   - b. rectifiers
   - c. polarity
   - d. wattage _____

10. The standard unit for measuring the _____ of an electric current is an ampere.
    a. volume   c. strength
    b. speed   d. density   _____

11. An ohm is used to measure the _____ of the current.
    a. resistance   c. volume
    b. strength   d. pressure   _____

12. A bulb that uses 40 watts of energy per second is a _____-watt bulb.
    a. 4   c. 400
    b. 40   d. 4000   _____

13. When the wire _____, a safety device called a fuse blows.
    a. suddenly shuts down
    b. becomes too hot from overloading the circuit
    c. blows up
    d. breaks in half   _____

14. _____ supply the same safety control as fuses.
    a. Plugs   c. Circuit breakers
    b. Grounds   d. GFCIs   _____

15. The influence that a charged body has _____ is called an electric field.
    a. over a conductor   c. on the space around it
    b. when wrapped in   d. on water
       an insulator   _____

16. Electrodes are commonly made of _____.
    a. carbon   c. silk
    b. silicon   d. metal   _____

17. Careful attention to electrical safety helps to eliminate accidental _____.
    a. shock   c. burns
    b. fire   d. All answers are correct.   _____

18. A cathode is a(n) _____.
    a. negative ion   c. negative electrode
    b. positive ion   d. positive electrode   _____

19. To determine the negative electrode, place the tips of two conducting cords _____.
    a. on two separate pieces of blue moistened litmus paper
    b. in a bowl of fresh water
    c. onto an electrode test strip
    d. None of the answers are correct.   _____

20. There are four main modalities, not including _____.
    a. galvanic   c. sinusoidal
    b. rheostat   d. faradic   _____

21. To soften tissues, use _____.
    a. negative polarity high-frequency current
    b. positive polarity high-frequency current
    c. positive polarity galvanic current
    d. negative polarity galvanic current   _____

22. Anaphoresis forces _____ into the tissues from the negative toward the positive pole.
    a. salt   c. sebum
    b. liquids   d. antiseptic   _____

23. A benefit of _____ current is increased blood circulation.
    a. anaphoresis   c. faradic
    b. modal   d. galvanic   _____

24. The _____ electrode is flat for Tesla high-frequency current.
    a. scalp   c. neck
    b. facial   d. hand   _____

25. Light waves produce _____, chemical reactions, or germicidal effects.
    a. electrical current   c. heat
    b. cellular damage   d. cooling   _____

26. Sixty-five percent of natural sunlight at the earth's surface is _____.
    a. ultraviolet   c. invisible
    b. infrared   d. visible   _____

27. Blue light _____.
    a. relieves pain
    b. relaxes muscles
    c. contains few heat rays
    d. should be used over creams or ointments   _____

28. Red light _____.
    a. should only be used on clean, bare skin
    b. produces the most heat
    c. contains all of the visible light of the spectrum
    d. produces chemical and germicidal effects   _____

29. UVB rays are the _____ rays in the middle of the
    UV range.
    a. tonic   c. most germicidal
    b. therapeutic   d. None of the answers
                                   are correct.   _____

30. Infrared rays _____.
    a. should be used for a minimum of 10 minutes
    b. can cause blistering
    c. produce no light whatsoever, only a rosy glow
       when active
    d. show up as red   _____

CHAPTER 10—PROPERTIES AND DISORDERS OF THE SKIN

Multiple Choice

1. Dermatology involves the scientific study of all of the following except the _____.
   - a. diseases of the skin
   - b. skin's function
   - c. skin's structure
   - d. cosmetic products used on skin
   _____

2. Skin with a smooth texture _____.
   - a. is healthy
   - b. needs chemical treatment to open up the pores
   - c. is too oily
   - d. None of the answers are correct.
   _____

3. Slight acidity of the skin indicates _____.
   - a. dehydration
   - b. poor diet
   - c. good health
   - d. that an acid-balanced face wash is required
   _____

4. The skin of the eyelids _____.
   - a. contains few blood vessels
   - b. is the thickest on the body
   - c. is a different color from the rest of the body
   - d. is the thinnest on the body
   _____

5. The skin is constructed of two clearly defined divisions: _____.
   - a. the epidermis and the dermis
   - b. the albinism and the dermis
   - c. the bromhidrosis and the epidermis
   - d. the collagen and the cicatrix
   _____

6. The strata are the layers of the _____.
   - a. cuticle
   - b. corium
   - c. epidermis
   - d. dermis
   _____

7. The stratum corneum consists of _____ cells that are continually shed and replaced by cells coming to the surface from the underlying layers.
   - a. infrequently spaced
   - b. tightly packed, scale-like
   - c. nerve and blood
   - d. collagen
   _____

8. The stratum granulosum consists of cells that look like _____.
   a. stars
   b. mucus
   c. scales
   d. distinct granules
   _____

9. The stratum spinosum is a sub-layer that lies above the _____ and beneath the granulosum.
   a. asteatosis
   b. basal strata
   c. bulla
   d. cutis
   _____

10. The _____ is also called the true skin.
    a. fissure
    b. elastin
    c. dermatitis
    d. dermis
    _____

11. The _____ is 25 times thicker than the epidermis.
    a. cyst
    b. melanin
    c. cuticle
    d. dermis
    _____

12. Papillae contain small structures called _____ with nerve fiber endings that are sensitive to touch and pressure.
    a. nevuses
    b. macules
    c. tactile corpuscles
    d. keloids
    _____

13. Hair follicles are found in the _____ layer of the dermis.
    a. basal
    b. papillary
    c. reticular
    d. clear
    _____

14. The reticular layer _____.
    a. contains melanin
    b. supplies the skin with oxygen and nutrients
    c. consists of adipose tissue
    d. is part of the epidermis
    _____

15. The subcutaneous tissue _____.
    a. gives smoothness and contour to the body
    b. is found in the epidermis
    c. contains sweat glands
    d. is the same thickness in all humans
    _____

16. Essential materials for growth, nourishment, and repair of the skin are supplied by lymph and _____.
    a. blood
    b. sweat
    c. sebum
    d. melanin
    _____

17. Networks of arteries and lymphatics in the _____ send their smaller branches to hair papillae, hair follicles, and skin glands.
    a. reticular layer
    b. subcutaneous tissue
    c. papillary layer
    d. None of the answers are correct.   _____

18. The sweat and _____ glands of the skin contain secretory nerve fibers.
    a. blood   c. oil
    b. lymph   d. fat   _____

19. Sensory nerve fibers _____.
    a. trigger goose bumps
    b. send messages to the brain
    c. regulate the excretion of perspiration
    d. regulate the excretion of sebum   _____

20. Motor nerve fibers _____.
    a. are distributed to the arrector pili muscles
    b. react to heat
    c. react to cold
    d. regulate the excretion of perspiration   _____

21. The nerve endings that provide the body with _____ are found in the papillary layer.
    a. messages from the brain
    b. the sense of touch
    c. the ability to form goose bumps
    d. All answers are correct.   _____

22. The _____ of skin is provided by elastin.
    a. elasticity and   c. texture
       flexibility   d. sense of touch
    b. color   _____

23. The primary source of _____ is melanin.
    a. skin elasticity   c. feeling in the skin
    b. skin color   d. blood supply to the skin _____

24. _____ is produced by melanosomes.
    a. Perspiration   c. Melanin
    b. Sensory nerve fiber   d. Sebum   _____

25. Sudoriferous glands are also known as _____ glands.
    a. sweat   c. sebaceous
    b. oil   d. follicle   _____

26. Sweat glands consist of a coiled base and a tube-like duct that terminates at the skin surface to form the _____.
    a. sweat pore   c. secretory nerve
    b. melanin   d. collagen   _____

27. The nervous system controls the _____.
    a. texture of the skin   c. color of the skin
    b. blood supply to the   d. excretion of sweat
       skin   _____

28. Sebum lubricates the skin and _____.
    a. protects it from germs
    b. preserves the softness of the hair
    c. helps the sensory nerves to feel
    d. All of the answers are correct.   _____

29. A blackhead is formed when _____ becomes hardened and the duct becomes blocked.
    a. elastin   c. collagen
    b. sweat   d. sebum   _____

30. One of the principal functions of the skin is _____.
    a. protection   c. respiration
    b. movement   d. reproduction   _____

31. Hypertrophies include _____ on the face or scalp.
    a. bruises   c. perspiration
    b. sebum   d. moles and warts   _____

32. _____ symptoms include burning.
    a. Subjective   c. Dermal
    b. Objective   d. None of the answers
                              are correct.   _____

33. Apply medicinal preparations _____.
    a. as you see fit
    b. as directed by the client
    c. as directed by a physician
    d. only when directed to by your supervisor   _____

34. A reaction _____ is an allergy.
    a. due to extreme sensitivity to normally harmless
       substances
    b. to poisonous substances
    c. to extremely acidic
    d. None of the answers are correct.   _____

35. Any condition or disease that makes a treatment or
    medication _____ is called a contraindication.
    a. optional   c. necessary
    b. recommended   d. inadvisable   _____

36. A disease that _____ is called an occupational disease.
    a. involves an allergy
    b. prevents you from working
    c. happens when you are at work
    d. results from contact associated with employment   _____

37. A disease that _____ is called a congenital disease.
    a. involves an allergy   c. is related to employment
    b. exists at birth   d. is always fatal   _____

38. _____ is a parasitic disease.
    a. Inflammation   c. An allergy
    b. Ringworm   d. A heart defect   _____

39. Disease that is _____ is seasonal.
    a. untreated by   c. influenced by the
       a doctor   weather
    b. allergic in nature   d. off and on again   _____

40. There are three types of _____: primary, secondary, and
    tertiary.
    a. allergies   c. subjective symptoms
    b. lesions   d. parasites   _____

41. A tumor is a(n) _____ lesion.
    a. primary   c. allergic
    b. secondary   d. pathogenic   _____

42. A ulcer is a(n) _____ lesion.
    a. fluid-filled   c. depressed
    b. above-the-skin   d. rounded   _____

43. Vesicles may be produced by _____.
    a. poison ivy and oak   c. cysts
    b. ulcers   d. bullas   _____

44. An excoriation may be formed by a _____.
    a. scale   c. scrape
    b. fissure   d. crust   _____

45. An example of a fissure is _____.
    a. a scrape   c. a discolored spot on
    b. chapped lips   the skin
                               d. a scab   _____

46. A keloid is a thick scar resulting from ____.
    a. excessive growth of fibrous tissue
    b. surgery
    c. a primary lesion
    d. a tumor

    _____

47. A mole is a small, spot or blemish on the skin ranging
    in color from ____.
    a. green to gray   c. pale tan to brown to
    b. pale tan to orange   bluish black
                              d. None of the answers are
                                 correct.

    _____

48. *Lentigines* is the technical term for ____.
    a. pimples   c. poison ivy
    b. freckles   d. a mole

    _____

49. *Nevus* is the technical term for a ____.
    a. mole   c. keloid
    b. wart   d. birth-mark

    _____

50. Anthrax is an inflammatory ____ skin disease
    characterized by the presence of a small, red-brown
    papule, followed by the formation of a pustule, vesicle,
    and hard swelling.
    a. viral   c. parasitic
    b. bacterial   d. None of the answers
                                 are correct.

    _____

51. Herpes simplex is a recurring ____ infection that
    produces fever blisters.
    a. bacterial   c. viral
    b. parasitic   d. fungal

    _____

52. Triggering factors for acne include ____.
    a. heredity   c. stress
    b. hormones   d. All of the answers
                                 are correct.

    _____

53. Grade ____ acne involves many closed comedones,
    increased numbers of open comedones, and increased
    numbers of papules and pustules.
    a. I   c. III
    b. II   d. IV

    _____

54. Comedones appear frequently on the ____.
    a. face   c. nose
    b. forehead   d. All answers are correct.

    _____

55. _____, dilation of the blood vessels, and the formation of papules and pustules characterizes rosacea.
    a. Pallor
    b. A gray skin tone
    c. Redness
    d. None of the answers are correct.   _____

56. A steatoma is a sebaceous cyst or _____ that is filled with sebum.
    a. fatty tumor
    b. ulcer
    c. comedone
    d. inflammation   _____

57. Exposure to excessive _____ may cause miliaria rubra.
    a. heat
    b. cold
    c. damp
    d. dryness   _____

58. Basal cell carcinoma is the _____.
    a. most severe form of skin cancer
    b. name for grade IV acne
    c. rarest type of skin cancer
    d. most common type of skin cancer   _____

59. _____ indicate squamous cell carcinoma.
    a. Light pearly nodules
    b. Scaly red papules or nodules
    c. Jagged patches
    d. Raised patches   _____

60. A well-balanced diet consists of _____ basic food groups.
    a. two
    b. three
    c. four
    d. five   _____

61. Vitamin C is important for _____.
    a. overall skin health
    b. rapid skin healing
    c. skin and tissue repair
    d. fighting the sun's effects   _____

62. Vitamin E helps to _____.
    a. eliminate toxins from the skin
    b. maintain moist skin
    c. heal the skin
    d. fight against the harmful effects of sunlight   _____

CHAPTER 11—PROPERTIES AND DISORDERS OF THE HAIR AND SCALP

Multiple Choice

1. *Trichos* is the Greek word for _____.
   - a. hair
   - b. beauty
   - c. beard
   - d. skin
   _____

2. One of the functions of hair is _____.
   - a. adornment
   - b. protecting the head from water
   - c. to show one's age
   - d. All of the answers are correct.
   _____

3. Hair and nails are composed of the same protein, _____.
   - a. keratin
   - b. papilla
   - c. catagen
   - d. canities
   _____

4. The main structures of the hair root are the follicle, bulb, dermal papilla, _____, and arrector pili muscle.
   - a. anagens
   - b. sebaceous glands
   - c. furuncles
   - d. eumelanin
   _____

5. The fewest number of hair follicles are found on the _____.
   - a. stomach and chest
   - b. face
   - c. palms of the hands and the soles of the feet
   - d. arms and legs
   _____

6. Each hair _____.
   - a. grows from a single follicle
   - b. may share the hair follicle with another
   - c. is set straight down into the skin
   - d. None of the answers are correct.
   _____

7. The mouths of hair follicles are _____.
   - a. funnel-shaped
   - b. star-shaped
   - c. round
   - d. scale-like
   _____

8. The dermal papilla is covered by the _____.
   - a. hair follicle
   - b. sebaceous gland
   - c. lower part of the hair bulb
   - d. upper part of the hair bulb
   _____

9. The dermal papilla _____.
   a. does not have any nerves
   b. is responsible for secreting sebum
   c. is responsible for new hair growth
   d. does not have a blood supply _____

10. A _____ is caused by the overproduction of sebum.
    a. common form of oily dandruff
    b. formation of scaly crusts
    c. healthy shine
    d. None of the answers are correct. _____

11. Sebum production is affected by _____.
    a. hair color   c. emotional
    b. weather   disturbances
                           d. location _____

12. The blood supply to the hair delivers _____.
    a. keratin   c. sebum
    b. nourishment   d. color _____

13. During adolescence, endocrine glands are very active;
    after _____, their activity usually decreases.
    a. childhood   c. middle age
    b. young adulthood   d. elderly adulthood _____

14. Eyebrow and eyelash hairs lack _____.
    a. follicles   c. blood supply
    b. keratin   d. arrector pili muscles _____

15. The cuticle is the _____ layer of the hair.
    a. outermost   c. middle
    b. innermost   d. thickest _____

16. The _____ of the hair consists of a single overlapping
    layer(s) of transparent, scale-like cells that point away
    from the scalp toward the hair ends.
    a. cuticle   c. medulla
    b. cortex   d. arrector _____

17. The cuticle is responsible for _____.
    a. hair color
    b. the shine and silkiness of the hair
    c. 90 percent of the hair's weight
    d. the strength and elasticity of hair _____

18. The cortex layer _____.
    a. is a single layer of cells
    b. accounts for most of the hair's weight
    c. is the outermost layer of the hair
    d. protects the hair from damage   _____

19. The _____ is the middle layer of the hair.
    a. cortex   c. medulla
    b. cuticle   d. pili   _____

20. The medulla is also called the _____ of the hair.
    a. pith   c. pith or marrow
    b. marrow   d. protein core   _____

21. Round cells make up the _____.
    a. medulla
    b. cuticle
    c. protein layer of the hair
    d. male beard   _____

22. Hair is composed of protein that grows from cells that
    originate within the _____.
    a. cuticle   c. cortex
    b. hair follicle   d. hair bed   _____

23. Twenty-one percent of hair is made of _____.
    a. carbon   c. nitrogen
    b. oxygen   d. sulfur   _____

24. _____ makes up 17 percent of hair.
    a. Carbon   c. Hydrogen
    b. Oxygen   d. Nitrogen   _____

25. _____ hair contains less carbon and more oxygen than
    other types.
    a. Light-colored   c. Curly
    b. Dark-colored   d. Straight   _____

26. The end-to-end bonds between amino acids are also
    called _____ bonds.
    a. peptide   c. peptide or end
    b. end   d. side   _____

27. The polypeptide chains intertwine around each other to
    create a coil or spiral of protein called a(n) _____.
    a. end-to-end bond   c. chain-link
    b. peptide bond   d. helix   _____

28. Barbers should be careful not to break _____ bonds with overprocessing.
   a. keratln
   b. amino
   c. end
   d. side

   _____

29. Millions of _____ are cross-linked to form a ladder-like structure.
   a. peptide bonds
   b. polypeptide chains
   c. end bonds
   d. side bonds

   _____

30. Salt bonds are broken by _____.
   a. water
   b. changes in pH
   c. heat
   d. thio perms

   _____

31. Disulfide bonds are broken by _____.
   a. water
   b. changes in pH
   c. hydroxide relaxers
   d. chemical depilatories

   _____

32. _____ bonds account for one-third of hair's total strength.
   a. Hydrogen
   b. Disulfide
   c. Salt
   d. All answers are correct.

   _____

33. Hydrogen bonds _____.
   a. allow hair to be curled using rollers
   b. are not easily broken by shampooing
   c. are strong covalent bonds
   d. are the least numerous

   _____

34. Strong acidic solutions easily break _____ bonds.
   a. salt
   b. hydrogen
   c. disulfide
   d. peptide

   _____

35. A sulfur bond is another name for a _____ bond.
   a. hydrogen
   b. salt
   c. disulfide
   d. peptide

   _____

36. There are two different types of melanin: eumelanin and _____.
   a. pheomelanin
   b. covalent
   c. disulfide
   d. medulla

   _____

37. The ratio of eumelanin to pheomelanin determines _____.
   a. hair density
   b. hair elasticity
   c. natural color
   d. hair strength

   _____

38. People with approximately 140,000 hairs on the head are _____
    a. black haired   c. redheads
    b. brown haired   d. blonde   _____

39. _____ have approximately 80,000 hairs on the head.
    a. Redheads   c. Black-haired people
    b. Blondes   d. Brown-haired people   _____

40. When describing the wave pattern of the hair, there are _____ standard choices.
    a. two   c. four
    b. three   d. five   _____

41. Round hair is found on people of _____ descent.
    a. Asian   c. African American
    b. Caucasian   d. Hispanic   _____

42. Hair is found all over the body except the _____.
    a. eyelids   c. lips
    b. palms   d. All answers are correct. _____

43. Vellus hair almost never has a _____.
    a. cuticle   c. medulla
    b. cortex   d. bulb   _____

44. Primary terminal hair grows on the _____.
    a. eyebrows and   c. scalp
       eyelashes   d. beard
    b. cheeks   _____

45. Secondary terminal hair replaces some _____ hair after puberty.
    a. curly   c. primary terminal
    b. straight   d. vellus   _____

46. When the follicles stop making terminal hair and revert back to producing the vellus type, _____ occurs.
    a. primary termination   c. male pattern baldness
    b. lanugo   d. puberty   _____

47. Between the ages of 15 and 30, _____.
    a. the growth rate for hair on the scalp slows
    b. the follicles on the scalp grow lanugo hair
    c. the growth of scalp hair occurs more rapidly
    d. the eyebrows and eyelashes grow vellus hair   _____

48. Hair growth is influenced by _____.
    a. hormones
    b. nutrition
    c. season
    d. All answers are correct.   _____

49. Losing 75 to 100 hairs per day is _____.
    a. lower than average
    b. normal
    c. higher than average
    d. cause for immediate
       concern   _____

50. A hair stream is _____.
    a. hair that flows in the same direction
    b. another name for curly hair
    c. another name for straight hair
    d. None of the answers are correct.   _____

51. During the anagen phase, _____.
    a. new hair is produced
    b. the follicle shrinks
    c. germ cells are grown
    d. the hair is shed   _____

52. The telogen phase is the _____ in the growth cycle.
    a. first
    b. second
    c. last
    d. longest   _____

53. Coarse hair _____.
    a. is the weakest
    b. has the smallest diameter
    c. is easily penetrated by chemicals
    d. is harder to penetrate using chemicals   _____

54. Wiry hair has a hard, glassy finish because the cuticle _____.
    a. is thicker
    b. is missing
    c. scales lie flat against the
       hair shaft
    d. scales point up   _____

55. Hair density of 2,200 strands per square inch is _____.
    a. very low
    b. somewhat low
    c. normal
    d. very high   _____

56. Hair with poor porosity _____.
    a. feels smooth
    b. is overly porous
    c. has been over-processed
    d. None of the answers
       are correct.   _____

58

57. The strength of the side bonds in the hair determines the hair's _____.
    a. porosity
    c. color
    b. elasticity
    d. density
    _____

58. Almost 40 percent of men and women show some degree of hair loss by age _____.
    a. 25
    c. 45
    b. 35
    d. 65
    _____

59. Alopecia senilis is the _____.
    a. normal loss of scalp hair occurring in old age
    b. premature loss of scalp hair
    c. hair loss that is a result of poor nutrition
    d. hair loss due to hormonal change
    _____

60. Finasteride is an oral prescription medication for men only sold under the brand name _____.
    a. Plugus
    c. Propeca
    b. Rogaine
    d. Minoxidil
    _____

61. Dandruff can be easily mistaken for _____ because the symptoms of both conditions are a flaky, itchy, irritated scalp.
    a. tinea
    c. malassezia
    b. dry scalp
    d. pediculosis
    _____

62. A fungus causes _____.
    a. dandruff
    c. folliculitis barbae
    b. pediculosis capitis
    d. pseudofolliculitis
    _____

63. A case of tinea usually starts with a(n) _____ that spread(s) outward and then heal(s) in the middle, with a scale-like appearance.
    a. inflamed pustule
    c. patch of scaly dry skin
    b. tender swollen area
    d. small, reddened patch of little blisters
    _____

64. _____ occurs in the beard.
    a. Dandruff
    c. Tinea sycosis
    b. Ringworm
    d. Carbuncles
    _____

65. _____ is the infestation of the hair and scalp with head lice.
    a. Scabies
    c. Pediculosis capitis
    b. Barber's itch
    d. Ringworm
    _____

66. Folliculitis can occur anywhere on the body as a result of _____ infection.
    - a. bacterial or viral
    - b. animal parasite
    - c. fungal
    - d. None of the answers are correct.

    _____

67. Improper shaving may cause _____.
    - a. pseudofolliculitis barbae
    - b. scabies
    - c. head lice
    - d. tinea sycosis

    _____

68. A carbuncle is similar to a _____ but is larger.
    - a. boil
    - b. sycosis barbae
    - c. furuncle
    - d. folliculitis

    _____

69. Disorders of the hair include _____.
    - a. pityriasis steatoide
    - b. tinea favosa
    - c. vulgaris
    - d. monilethrix

    _____

70. _____ hair is a form of canities.
    - a. Gray
    - b. Knotted
    - c. Curly
    - d. Ringed

    _____

71. *Trichorrhexis nodosa* is the technical term for _____ hair.
    - a. ringed
    - b. knotted
    - c. gray
    - d. white

    _____

CHAPTER 12—TREATMENT OF THE HAIR AND SCALP

Multiple Choice

1. Shampoo is the best product to _____.
   - a. replenish protein in the hair
   - b. style the hair
   - c. moisturize the hair
   - d. clean the hair and scalp

   _____

2. Volumizing shampoo is ideal for _____ hair.
   - a. straight, fine
   - b. coarse
   - c. dry
   - d. curly

   _____

3. Moisturizing shampoo is a good choice for _____ hair.
   - a. straight, fine
   - b. damaged
   - c. wavy or curly
   - d. dry

   _____

4. Dry and damaged hair benefits from _____.
   - a. acid-balanced shampoo
   - b. leave-in conditioner
   - c. volumizing shampoo
   - d. deep-conditioning treatments

   _____

5. Chair cloths are also called _____.
   - a. haircutting capes
   - b. neck cloths
   - c. shampoo capes
   - d. nylon capes

   _____

6. Before draping the client, you should _____.
   - a. make an appointment for the next service
   - b. sanitize your hands
   - c. perform the client consultation
   - d. shampoo the client's hair

   _____

7. When draping for wet hair services, place the towel _____.
   - a. around the back of the neck only
   - b. across the chin in the front
   - c. lengthwise around the client's neck
   - d. widthwise around the client's neck

   _____

8. When performing chemical services, _____.
   - a. place one towel under the cape only
   - b. place one towel under and one over the cape
   - c. place one towel under and two over the cape
   - d. None of the answers are correct.

   _____

9. While performing the shampoo, the barber _____.
   - a. puts on his waterproof jacket
   - b. stands behind the shampoo bowl
   - c. stands beside the client
   - d. sits down

   _____

10. To maintain good posture while shampooing, _____.
    a. keep the knees locked
    b. stand as far as possible from the client's head
    c. lean as far forward as possible
    d. keep the abdomen flat   _____

11. When choosing a shampoo product, consider _____
    characteristics of the hair and scalp.
    a. three   c. five
    b. four   d. six   _____

12. The barber should consider the _____ when choosing
    products.
    a. condition of the hair   c. hair color
    b. hair length   d. hair's wave pattern   _____

13. Shampoo should be dispensed into the barber's hand,
    then _____.
    a. spread over the barber's palms
    b. onto the top of the client's head
    c. onto the back of the client's head
    d. onto the client's hand   _____

14. When shampooing, remove excess lather _____.
    a. with the fingertips   c. with a strong spray
    b. with a sweep of   d. using a lather brush
       the palm   _____

15. During a shampoo service, massage the scalp _____.
    a. before applying shampoo
    b. immediately after applying shampoo
    c. after rinsing out the shampoo
    d. after applying conditioner   _____

16. A piece of cotton is used to apply _____ shampoo.
    a. liquid-dry   c. dry
    b. regular shampoo   d. powder   _____

17. When the client's health will not permit a wet shampoo,
    _____ shampoo is used.
    a. liquid-dry   c. conditioning
    b. dry   d. All of the answers
                                   are correct.   _____

18. The scalp steam is effective in _____.
    a. preparing the scalp for scalp massage manipulations
       and treatments
    b. providing an alternative to shampoo
    c. closing the pores
    d. None of the answers are correct.   _____

19. When performing scalp massage, apply _____ pressure on the upward strokes.
    a. no
    b. little
    c. firm
    d. soft
    _____

20. Place the hands at the hairline to _____.
    a. finish a scalp massage
    b. begin a scalp massage
    c. begin shampooing the hair
    d. apply liquid-dry shampoo
    _____

21. During scalp massage, the neck-to-crown movement affects the _____ muscle.
    a. auricularis posterior
    b. frontalis
    c. auricularis superior
    d. auricularis anterior
    _____

22. During a scalp massage, the temporal auricular nerve is affected by the _____ movement.
    a. neck-to-crown
    b. forehead-to-crown
    c. ear-to-crown
    d. sliding
    _____

23. During general scalp treatment, _____ is an optional step.
    a. massaging the hair
    b. hair and scalp analysis
    c. infrared treatment
    d. applying high-frequency current
    _____

24. _____ contributes to dry hair and scalp.
    a. Overactivity of the oil glands
    b. Removal of natural oil
    c. An indoor lifestyle
    d. Infrequent washing
    _____

25. Overactive sebaceous glands cause _____.
    a. a dry scalp
    b. an oily scalp
    c. glossy hair
    d. decreased circulation
    _____

26. _____ of the scalp may contribute to dandruff.
    a. Excessive perspiration
    b. Sunlight exposure
    c. Overactive oil production
    d. Poor blood circulation
    _____

27. The technical term for hair loss is _____.
    a. antidandruff
    b. alopecia
    c. emollient
    d. sebaceous
    _____

28. Treatment for the hair shaft is called a(n) _____ treatment.
    a. corrective hair
    b. infrared
    c. high frequency
    d. tonic
    _____

CHAPTER 13—MEN'S FACIAL MASSAGE AND TREATMENTS

Multiple Choice

1. About 20 percent of the skin care clientele in spas and salons is _____.
   - a. over age 50
   - b. under age 50
   - c. female
   - d. male
   _____

2. Regularly scheduled facials produce noticeable improvement in all of the areas except _____.
   - a. skin tone
   - b. skin texture
   - c. skin appearance
   - d. skin color
   _____

3. There are three _____ systems associated with the performance of facial treatments.
   - a. full body
   - b. subdermal
   - c. external
   - d. epidermal
   _____

4. Arteries are _____ blood vessels that transport blood under very high pressure.
   - a. elastic
   - b. muscular
   - c. thick-walled
   - d. All answers are correct.
   _____

5. Muscular tissue may be stimulated using all of the following except _____.
   - a. massage
   - b. electric current
   - c. hair
   - d. visible light rays
   _____

6. The aponeurosis muscle is located in the _____.
   - a. scalp
   - b. shoulders
   - c. neck
   - d. cheek
   _____

7. The procerus _____.
   - a. covers the top of the skull
   - b. causes wrinkles across the bridge of the nose
   - c. compresses the cheeks
   - d. draws the corner of the mouth out and back
   _____

8. The corrugator affects the _____.
   - a. eyebrows
   - b. mouth
   - c. cheeks
   - d. forehead
   _____

9. The _____ muscles are the masseter and the temporalis.
   - a. skull
   - b. mastication
   - c. lip
   - d. ear
   _____

10. The trapezius _____.
    a. is located in the nose area
    b. draws down the corner of the mouth
    c. is responsible for depressing the lower jar
    d. covers the back of the neck   _____

11. There are 12 pairs of _____ nerves and all are connected
    to a part of the brain surface.
    a. arterial   c. spinal
    b. cranial   d. cervical   _____

12. The third cranial nerve controls the _____.
    a. motion of the eye   c. sensations of the face
    b. sense of smell   d. motions of the face   _____

13. The trifacial is a _____ nerve.
    a. sensory   c. sensory-motor
    b. motor   d. cervical   _____

14. The _____ nerve controls the motion of the eye.
    a. vagus   c. optic
    b. olfactory   d. abducent   _____

15. The vagus nerve controls the _____.
    a. sense of hearing
    b. sensations of the larynx
    c. motion of the tongue
    d. upward motion of the eye   _____

16. The seventh cranial nerve includes the _____ nerve.
    a. acoustic   c. supraorbital
    b. trochlear   d. posterior auricular   _____

17. The _____ nerves include the olfactory nerve.
    a. sensory   c. sensory-motor
    b. motor   d. cervical   _____

18. The greater occipital nerve is located _____.
    a. at the back of the head
    b. at the base of the skull
    c. on the left side of the neck
    d. on the right side of the neck   _____

19. The greater auricular nerve affects the _____.
    a. scalp   c. external ears
    b. top of the head   d. front of the neck   _____

20. _____ is/are not part of the circulatory system.
    a. Nerves   c. Arteries
    b. Blood   d. Veins   _____

21. The common carotids _____.
    a. are the main sources of blood supply to the head,
       face, and neck
    b. include the submental branch
    c. supply the masseter
    d. supply the skin in back of the ear   _____

22. The occipital artery supplies the _____.
    a. front, side, and top of the head
    b. sternocleidomastoideus muscle
    c. scalp and back of the head up to the crown
    d. ear   _____

23. There are _____ principal veins in the neck.
    a. one   c. three
    b. two   d. four   _____

24. Normal skin can receive _____ massage.
    a. soothing   c. strongly stimulating
    b. mildly stimulating   d. All answers are correct. _____

25. _____ is a condition that precludes massage.
    a. Slightly inflamed skin c. Recent exercise
    b. High blood pressure   d. Dry skin   _____

26. When applying _____ manipulations, pressure
    should be applied on the upward swing of the
    movement.
    a. rhythmic   c. motor point
    b. clockwise   d. rotary   _____

27. A motor point is a(n) _____, where pressure or
    stimulation will cause contraction of a muscle.
    a. point on a nerve   c. joint
    b. point on the skin,   d. artery or vein
       over a muscle   _____

28. Effleurage is a _____ that should be applied in a
    slow and rhythmic manner over the skin with no
    pressure.
    a. short, quick slapping c. light, continuous
       motion   movement
    b. strong rubbing   d. tapping movement   _____

29. The palms are used to perform effleurage _____.
      a. if the fingertips   c. on large surfaces
         are sore   d. only on the face
      b. on small surfaces

_____

30. During pétrissage, the skin and flesh are _____.
      a. grasped between the thumb and fingers
      b. stroked gently
      c. massaged deeply using the fists
      d. rapidly vibrated using the fingers

_____

31. Friction has proven beneficial to the _____ of the skin.
      a. texture and color   c. loosening and flexibility
      b. toning   d. circulation and
                                    glandular activity

_____

32. Percussion is the most _____ type of massage.
      a. stimulating   c. uncomfortable
      b. relaxing   d. None of the answers
                                    are correct.

_____

33. The tapping movement of _____ can be used in facial massage.
      a. effleurage   c. percussion
      b. vibration   d. friction

_____

34. Vibration is a type of massage that can be formed with _____.
      a. the palms   c. an electric massager
      b. a massage chair   d. an electrode

_____

35. After a massage, the skin _____.
      a. decreases functional activities
      b. increases functional activities
      c. feels cold to the touch
      d. becomes very sensitive

_____

36. _____ is a benefit of massage.
      a. Smoothing of muscle   c. Reduced need for
         fibers   blood circulation
      b. Reduction of fat cells d. Excitement of nerves

_____

37. When massaging the nose, _____.
      a. stroke upward
      b. use a circular motion
      c. move the nose from side to side
      d. None of the answers are correct.

_____

38. The final part of the face to be massaged is the _____.
    a. forehead
    b. nose
    c. around the yes
    d. neck
    _____

39. The brush machine helps to _____ the skin.
    a. stimulate
    b. cleanse
    c. lightly exfoliate
    d. All answers are correct.
    _____

40. When using a brush machine on oily skin, use _____.
    a. a higher speed
    b. a lower speed
    c. the exfoliation setting
    d. no pressure
    _____

41. To prepare steam towels, fold the towel lengthwise and then in half, then _____.
    a. pour witch hazel on the towel
    b. place the towel in the cabinet
    c. run hot water over the towel
    d. run warm water over the towel
    _____

42. Sinus conditions and congestion can be improved with _____.
    a. a steamer
    b. a brush machine
    c. drinking distilled water
    d. an electric massager.
    _____

43. _____ rays are used to produce different effects through the use of therapeutic lamps.
    a. Microwave
    b. Gamma
    c. Green and yellow
    d. Infrared and ultraviolet
    _____

44. A positive electrode is red with a _____.
    a. plus sign
    b. minus sign
    c. diamond shape
    d. black outline
    _____

45. High-frequency machine electrodes are made of glass or _____.
    a. plastic
    b. rubber
    c. metal
    d. wood
    _____

46. Tesla high-frequency current should not be used on clients who _____.
    a. suffer from hair loss
    b. suffer from seizures
    c. have low blood pressure
    d. have had a cold in the past month
    _____

47. During facial treatment with high-frequency current, use the _____ electrode.
    a. rake
    b. flat
    c. mushroom-shaped
    d. negative
    _____

48. During indirect application of high-frequency current, the barber _____ the client's forehead.
   a. places the fingers of one hand on
   c. massages
   d. brushes
   b. places both palms on

49. Desincrustation is used to facilitate _____.
   a. deep pore cleansing
   b. cleaning
   c. blood circulation
   d. calming of the nerves

50. During the desincrustation procedure, the electrode is dipped in _____ and then applied to the client's forehead.
   a. acid-based solution
   b. alkaline solution
   c. water
   d. oil

51. Products that have a slightly acid pH are considered _____.
   a. neutral
   b. harmful
   c. positive
   d. negative

52. The microdermabrasion machine is a(n) _____ that is used to spray micro-crystals across the skin's surface through a closed stainless steel or glass pressurized wand.
   a. high-frequency current
   b. electronic vacuum
   c. brush
   d. electrode

53. White light _____.
   a. increases the elimination of waste products
   b. heats and relaxes the skin
   c. relieves pain in the back of the neck and shoulders
   d. improves dry skin

54. Cleansing is considered a _____ treatment.
   a. preservative
   b. hygienic
   c. corrective
   d. subdermal

55. The stimulation of _____ and protection of the skin surface are the objectives of a facial treatment for dry skin.
   a. blood circulation
   b. lymph circulation
   c. oil production
   d. sweat production

56. Face washes are usually water-based products with a _____ pH effective on oily and combination skin types.
   a. neutral or slightly acidic
   b. strongly acidic
   c. strongly alkaline
   d. neutral or slightly alkaline

57. Astringents may contain up to _____ percent alcohol and are used for oily and acne-prone skin.
    a. 20
    b. 30
    c. 35
    d. 45 _____

58. Paraffin melts at _____.
    a. over 110 degrees
    b. 110 degrees
    c. slightly more than body temperature
    d. body temperature _____

59. Another name for the _____ facial is the scientific rest facial.
    a. corrective
    b. basic
    c. men's
    d. rolling cream _____

60. The first step in performing a basic facial is _____.
    a. adjusting the chair to recline
    b. product selection
    c. skin analysis
    d. draping _____

61. During a basic facial, a spatula is used _____.
    a. for massage
    b. during washing the face
    c. to remove products from containers
    d. to apply products _____

62. During a basic facial, apply steam towels _____.
    a. after exfoliation
    b. after the massage
    c. after applying and removing cleansing cream
    d. before cleansing cream _____

63. During a basic facial, avoid _____.
    a. a rough massage
    b. warm towels
    c. a stimulating massage
    d. gossiping with the client _____

64. When performing a(n) _____ facial, delicate areas around the nose and upper cheek require a special technique using both of the barber's hands.
    a. vibratory
    b. brush machine
    c. basic
    d. effleurage _____

65. During a vibratory facial, the _____ is massaged with slow, light strokes.
    a. forehead
    b. cheek
    c. temple
    d. nose _____

66. _____ is not a reason to avoid vibratory massage.
    a. Weakness of the   c. Skin inflammation
       heart   d. Sinus congestion
    b. Fever
    _____

67. _____ cream is used during a vibratory massage.
    a. Cleansing   c. Massage
    b. Exfoliating   d. Moisturizing
    _____

68. The rolling cream facial _____.
    a. is currently the most popular type of facial for men
    b. is recommended only for clients with dry skin
    c. is never performed any more
    d. was once most often identified with the barbershop
    _____

69. During a rolling cream facial, the cream is spread over the face with _____.
    a. a spatula   c. dampened fingers
    b. the palms   d. dry fingers
    _____

70. During a(n) _____ facial, apply lubricating oil over and under the eyes.
    a. ultraviolet   c. galvanic current
    b. infrared ray   d. oily skin
    _____

71. Do not permit infrared rays to remain on the body tissues for more than a few seconds at a time by _____.
    a. moving your hand back and forth across the rays' path
    b. using a patch to block the rays
    c. using lubricating oil
    d. turning the machine off every few seconds
    _____

72. During a facial that uses galvanic current, apply negative galvanic current for 5 to 7 minutes to _____.
    a. stimulate the nerves   c. close the pores
    b. soften the skin   d. open the pores
    _____

73. During a procedure with galvanic current, the _____ closes the pores.
    a. negative current   c. massage cream
    b. positive current   d. rolling cream
    _____

74. Indirect high-frequency current should be applied for _____ minutes.
    a. 1 to 2   c. 5 to 7
    b. 3 to 4   d. 7 to 10
    _____

75. During a facial for oily skin, analyze the skin under a magnifying lamp after _____.
    a. applying and removing cleansing lotion
    b. draping
    c. applying massage cream
    d. using a toner or astringent   _____

76. During a facial for acne, a high-frequency current may be applied for _____.
    a. 30 seconds   c. up to 5 minutes
    b. up to 1 minute   d. up to 10 minutes   _____

77. The hot-oil mask can be used for _____ skin that is prevalent during dry, hot, or windy weather.
    a. extremely dry   c. scaly
    b. parched   d. All answers are correct.   _____

78. A hot-oil mask is made with olive and _____ oil.
    a. castor   c. vegetable
    b. walnut   d. corn   _____

CHAPTER 14—SHAVING AND FACIAL HAIR DESIGN

Multiple Choice

1. Professional barbers use a straight razor of the changeable blade or _____ type when shaving a client.
   a. conventional
   b. disposable
   c. safety
   d. electric

   _____

2. Protective gloves are _____ while shaving a client.
   a. always optional
   b. required by some states
   c. always required
   d. unnecessary

   _____

3. Nicks or cuts are treated with styptic powder applied using a _____.
   a. bare finger
   b. cotton swab
   c. gloved finger
   d. tissue

   _____

4. Always use a light touch and a forward gliding motion that leads with the _____.
   a. side of the razor
   b. back of the razor
   c. point of the blade
   d. front of the blade

   _____

5. Always observe the hair growth pattern and _____.
   a. use more or less lather as required
   b. advise the client if shaving is advised
   c. shave with it, not against it
   d. shave against it rather than with it

   _____

6. When shaving a client, use the cushions of the fingertips to _____.
   a. apply lather to the area about to be shaved
   b. hold the client's chin steady
   c. stretch skin in the opposite direction of the razor stroke
   d. stretch skin in the same direction as the razor stroke

   _____

7. Improper shaving of curly hair can result in _____.
   a. acne
   b. too close a shave
   c. infected bumps on and under the skin surface
   d. an itchy rash

   _____

8. Barbers should be especially careful when shaving _____ to avoid irritation or injury.
   a. the upper neck
   b. around the sideburns
   c. beneath the lower lip
   d. the tops of the cheeks _____

9. When holding the razor, the little finger _____ the razor.
   a. guides
   b. does not touch
   c. balances
   d. braces _____

10. The term *cutting stroke* describes the _____.
    a. way the razor is held in the fingers
    b. position of the razor perpendicular to the floor
    c. correct angle of cutting with a razor
    d. correct direction of cutting with a razor _____

11. _____ refers to the way the razor is held in the barber's hand to facilitate a technique or stroke movement.
    a. Cutting stroke
    b. Position
    c. Razor stroke
    d. Hold _____

12. The client's skin is stretched with the _____ and second finger.
    a. first
    b. thumb
    c. third
    d. fourth _____

13. Very fast and very slow razor movements _____.
    a. are ideal for shaving all areas
    b. should be avoided
    c. are ideal for shaving some areas
    d. should only be used on the cheeks _____

14. Working efficiently and effectively includes all of the following *except* _____.
    a. leaving a small portion of lather behind for the next stroke
    b. making strokes so that no lather is left behind
    c. keeping the non-dominant hand dry for stretching purposes
    d. checking work for missed patches _____

15. The _____ stroke is employed at the sideburn and behind the ear areas during neck and outline shaves.
    a. reverse backhand
    b. freehand
    c. backhand
    d. reverse freehand _____

16. For the _____ stroke, the razor should be held with the handle between the third and fourth fingers.
    a. free finger
    b. reverse backhand
    c. freehand
    d. backhand _____

17. When shaving in the freehand position, _____.
    a. use a gliding stroke away from you
    b. use a gliding stroke toward you
    c. hold the razor in the left hand if you are right-handed
    d. rest the small finger on the shank of the razor near the shoulder of the blade _____

18. The _____ position and stroke is used in 6 of the 14 shaving areas.
    a. backhand
    b. freehand
    c. reverse freehand
    d. reverse backhand _____

19. For the freehand position, the _____ of the razor is held between the thumb and first two fingers.
    a. blade
    b. edge
    c. shank
    d. None of the answers are correct. _____

20. The _____ stroke is used in of the 14 basic shaving areas and if preferred in area 12.
    a. backhand
    b. freehand
    c. reverse freehand
    d. reverse backhand _____

21. When performing the reverse freehand stroke, the barber stands _____.
    a. behind the client's head
    b. to the client's left
    c. to the client's right
    d. facing the client _____

22. When using the reverse backhand stroke, employ a _____ stroke that follows along the natural hairline.
    a. sideways gliding
    b. circular
    c. upward gliding
    d. downward gliding _____

23. In the _____ position, turn the palm of the right hand to the right so that it faces upward.
    a. reverse backhand
    b. reverse freehand
    c. freehand
    d. backhand _____

24. For a right-handed barber, the backhand stroke is used to shave the _____.
    a. right sideburn
    b. right side below the jaw
    c. left sideburn
    d. right side of the neck _____

25. For a right-handed barber, the freehand or backhand stroke may be used to shave the _____.
   a. mlddle of the neck   c. right sideburn
   b. left side of the neck   d. area below the chin   _____

26. The reverse freehand position is used to shave the _____.
   a. middle of the neck   c. left upper lip
   b. right upper lip   d. left side below the jaw   _____

27. Lay a towel diagonally across the client's chest _____.
   a. before draping   c. to prepare for a shave
      the client   d. after drying the hair
   b. after shaving the client   _____

28. To cool an excessively hot steam towel, _____.
   a. put it in a refrigerator
   b. let the folded towel sit on the counter
   c. hold it by the top corners and fan it back and forth
   d. unfold it fully and spread it over an unused barber chair   _____

29. Do not use a hot steam towel if the skin is _____.
   a. sensitive   c. wrinkled
   b. dry   d. oily   _____

30. Immediately before applying lather, _____.
   a. remove the steam   c. wash your hands
      towel   d. None of the answers
   b. wash the face   are correct.   _____

31. Rubbing time for lather is from the 1 to 2 minutes, depending on the _____.
   a. client's preference   c. stiffness and density
   b. barber's preference   of the beard
      d. amount of lather   _____

32. The ideal razor movement is a _____ motion.
   a. sawing   c. sideways
   b. scraping   d. gliding

33. When shaving area No. 1, shave from the right sideburn to the _____.
   a. top of the right cheek   c. right side of the nose
   b. corner of the mouth   d. right side of the chin   _____

34. Shaving area No. _____ requires a freehand stroke starting at the chin.
    a. 4   c. 6
    b. 5   d. 7   _____

35. When the hair in shaving area No. 5 grows _____, the freehand stroke may be a better choice than the reverse freehand stroke.
    a. in whorls   c. downward
    b. sideways   d. upward   _____

36. When shaving area No. _____, the barber stands to the client's right.
    a. 7   c. 10
    b. 8   d. 11   _____

37. In shaving areas _____, the client can help to stretch the skin if he rolls his bottom lip slightly over his bottom teeth.
    a. 2 and 3   c. 10 and 12
    b. 5 and 7   d. 11 and 14   _____

38. Shaving area No. 13 includes the _____.
    a. left sideburn   c. chin
    b. right sideburn   d. Adam's apple   _____

39. After a shave, do not use _____.
    a. warm towels   c. hot towels
    b. facial cream   d. moisturizer   _____

40. _____ and witch hazel are astringent preparations commonly used in the barbershop.
    a. Exfoliants   c. Aftershave lotion
    b. Scrubs   d. High-pH astringents   _____

41. Towel wraps are used for _____.
    a. massage
    b. removing blackheads
    c. applying powder to the face
    d. All of the answers are correct.   _____

42. Complete outline shaves _____.
    a. are part of standard shaving
    b. accompany a facial
    c. typically follow a haircut
    d. are not performed by regular barbers   _____

43. After shaving the neck, _____.
    a. suggest a haircut
    b. shampoo the client's hair
    c. shave the beard
    d. suggest a leave-in scalp treatment _____

44. Large facial features do well with a _____ mustache.
    a. heavier looking
    b. narrow
    c. semi-square
    d. pyramid-shaped _____

45. A _____ looks best with a semi-square mustache.
    a. face with an extra-small mouth
    b. long, narrow
    c. round face with regular features
    d. face with small features _____

46. Use a _____ or outliner to shape the mustache.
    a. razor
    b. shears
    c. trimmer
    d. mustache shaper _____

47. Gently comb the beard _____.
    a. right after consulting with the client about beard design
    b. before draping the client
    c. after performing a neck shave
    d. None of the answers are correct. _____

CHAPTER 15—MEN'S HAIRCUTTING AND STYLING

Multiple Choice

1. During the client consultation, the barber should _____.
   a. analyze the client's hair and scalp
   b. shampoo the client's hair
   c. schedule the next appointment
   d. All of the above.   _____

2. When the barber asks the client how long it has been since his last haircut, he is trying to determine _____.
   a. the client's income
   b. how frequently he will see the client for scheduling purposes
   c. the client's hair growth rate
   d. the texture of the client's hair   _____

3. Envisioning is the process of _____ based on what the client has told you.
   a. describing the client's ideal haircut
   b. picturing or visualizing in your mind the finished cut and style
   c. determining the specific length of the hair that will be cut
   d. None of the answers are correct.   _____

4. The facial _____ of each individual is determined by the position and prominence of the facial bones.
   a. size   c. tone
   b. shape   d. All of the answers
                                 are correct.   _____

5. A round face benefits from _____.
   a. extra height on top   c. wavy bangs
   b. hair close to   d. a layered cut
      the crown   _____

6. A square face looks good with _____.
   a. an off-center part
   b. wavy bangs that blend into the temples
   c. a square beard
   d. a mustache that shortens the face   _____

7. Concave profiles require _____.
   a. a beard or goatee
   b. a lot of height at the top of the head
   c. a close hair arrangement over the forehead
   d. almost any hairstyle   _____

8. A straight profile tends to be the most balanced and _____.
   a. can usually wear any hairstyle successfully
   b. requires blown bangs over the forehead
   c. looks better with a mustache only
   d. looks best with a beard only _____

9. Prominent nose shapes include hooked, _____, and large noses.
   a. small
   b. medium
   c. turned-up
   d. pointed _____

10. Reference points are points on the head that mark areas where the surface of the head changes or the behavior of the hair changes _____.
    a. as a result of curly hair
    b. due to differing hair density
    c. due to different hair textures
    d. as a result of the surface changes _____

11. The _____ is also known as the crest, temporal, horseshoe, or hatband area of the head.
    a. apex
    b. crown
    c. occipital bone
    d. parietal ridge _____

12. The occipital bone protrudes _____.
    a. at the base of the skull
    b. on the top of the head
    c. at the widest part of the head
    d. None of the answers are correct. _____

13. Horizontal lines are usually created at the perimeter or at the _____ of a haircut.
    a. apex
    b. crest
    c. occipital area
    d. nape _____

14. Vertical lines facilitate _____ while cutting.
    a. the use of blunt layers
    b. the projection of the hair at higher elevations
    c. creating a one-length cut
    d. All of the answers are correct. _____

15. Diagonal lines may be used to create a _____ effect at the perimeter or to blend longer layers to shorter layers within a haircut.
    a. horizontal
    b. blunt
    c. curved
    d. stacked layered _____

16. Angles help to create strong, consistent _____ in haircutting.
    a. layers
    b. foundations
    c. outlines
    d. projections _____

17. Zero elevation means that the hair is _____.
    a. is not lifted at all
    b. is held perpendicular to the floor
    c. is held parallel to the floor
    d. is lifted straight from the roots _____

18. Use of a vertical parting projected at 45 degrees, with the fingers holding the parting angled at a _____, will create a tapered effect.
    a. 30-degree diagonal
    b. 45-degree diagonal
    c. 60-degree angle
    d. 90-degree angle _____

19. A 90-degree elevation is used to create _____.
    a. medium elevation
    b. a stationary guide
    c. uniform layers
    d. a perimeter line _____

20. _____ or partings are used to create subsections to gain control of the hair while cutting.
    a. Parts
    b. Elevations
    c. Parings
    d. Guides _____

21. The cutting line refers to the _____.
    a. depth of the part from the apex
    b. elevation of the hair
    c. position of the fingers when cutting a section of hair
    d. position of the shears when cutting a section of hair _____

22. _____ are classified as being either stationary or traveling.
    a. Cutting lines
    b. Guides
    c. Elevations
    d. Projections _____

23. Uniform layers are _____.
    a. even throughout
    b. shorter on top
    c. longer on top
    d. the same length at the bottom _____

24. A weight line refers to the _____.
    a. heaviest perimeter area of a 45-elevation or 0-degree cut
    b. heaviest perimeter area of a 0-elevation or 45-degree cut
    c. lightest perimeter area of a 45-elevation or 0-degree cut
    d. lightest perimeter area of a 0-elevation or 45-degree cut
    _____

25. Use maximum tension on _____.
    a. curly hair to create uniform layers
    b. curly hair to create even length
    c. curly hair to create precise lines
    d. straight hair to create precise lines
    _____

26. Thinning refers to _____.
    a. tapering the angle of a cut
    b. removing excess bulk from the hair
    c. evening out a blunt cut
    d. adding long layers to remove height
    _____

27. Cutting above the fingers is frequently used in men's haircutting to cut and blend layers in the _____ area.
    a. top   c. horseshoe
    b. crown   d. All answers are correct.
    _____

28. Cutting below the fingers is most often used to create design lines at the _____.
    a. apex   c. horseshoe area
    b. nape of the neck   d. perimeter of the haircut
    _____

29. When using the _____ technique, both the fingers and comb should be in a horizontal position parallel to the floor.
    a. thinning   c. comb-and-shear
    b. projection   d. fingers-and-shear
    _____

30. The standard fingers-and-shear cutting method should be used for all hair types *except* _____ hair.
    a. moderately thick   c. curly
    b. excessively bristly   d. dry
    _____

31. The _____ cutting technique is normally performed in the nape.
    a. shear-over-fingers   c. fingers-over-comb
    b. comb-over-shear   d. shear-over-comb
    _____

32. When using the shear-over-comb technique, place the third finger _____.
     a. so that it does not touch the shears
     c. on the shank of the comb
     b. into the finger grip
     d. on the finger brace _____

33. In the shear-over-comb technique, the comb is held in the left hand with the fingers on top of the teeth and the thumb _____.
     a. on the finger grip of the shear
     b. on the backbone of the comb
     c. on the brace of the shear
     d. alongside the fingers _____

34. In the shear-over-comb technique, align the still blade of the shears with the comb _____.
     a. at the top of the backbone
     b. below the still blade
     c. at the level where the teeth join the back
     d. None of the answers are correct. _____

35. The arching technique can be used to thin _____.
     a. hollows
     c. whorls
     b. wrinkles
     d. All answers are correct. _____

36. When using the arching technique, the barber _____.
     a. starts behind the ear
     b. does not modify the shape of the sideburn
     c. gently tugs the client's ear down
     d. uses the center of the shear blade _____

37. The standard techniques for clipper cutting are _____ cutting and clipper-over-comb cutting.
     a. freehand clipper
     c. clipper and razor
     b. shear-over-clipper
     d. clipper outlining _____

38. When tight, curly hair is cut _____, the clipper blade gets clogged and patches and spots may be left.
     a. with a short blade
     c. against the grain
     b. with the grain
     d. using clipper guides _____

39. Many barbers prefer to use an outliner or trimmer with a fine cutting edge to _____.
     a. cut at the apex
     c. form the cutting line
     b. square off sideburns
     d. form the design line _____

40. Very short curly hair requires true _____ clipper cutting technique.
    a. freehand
    b. shorthand
    c. clipper-over-comb
    d. None of the answers are correct.
    _____

41. Size 0000 detachable blades are _____.
    a. closest to shaving
    b. no longer used
    c. dangerous because they can cut the client
    d. the longest size
    _____

42. When using the clipper-over-comb cutting technique, the _____ is placed on the top left side of the clipper
    a. thumb
    b. index finger
    c. middle finger
    d. pinky
    _____

43. Begin in the nape area _____.
    a. only when using an adjustable blade clipper
    b. for very short hair
    c. only when using 0000 blades
    d. for freehand clipper cutting
    _____

44. Short styles, such as _____, have a high taper and are blended in the crest areas.
    a. butch
    b. crew cuts
    c. fades
    d. All answers are correct.
    _____

45. Flat tops are traditionally slightly longer in the _____ sections and flat across the top of the head form.
    a. front and crest
    b. front and nape
    c. side and back
    d. side and bottom
    _____

46. A brush cut is also called a _____.
    a. flat top
    b. crew cut
    c. Quo Vadis
    d. military cut
    _____

47. The Quo Vadis is a popular very short haircut style that is suitable for _____ hair.
    a. very curly
    b. curly
    c. somewhat curly
    d. straight
    _____

48. Long haircut styles usually require the least amount of _____.
    a. work with the shears
    b. time
    c. comb work
    d. clipper tapering
    _____

49. When performing a _____ cut, clipper cutting in the nape should be performed with the clipper tilted on its heel until reaching a point about midway to the ears.
    a. brush
    b. medium length
    c. long
    d. Quo Vadis

50. In a _____ style, when cutting around the ears, remove about 1 inch from the hairline, then use an outliner to trim the sideburns and around the ear areas.
    a. short
    b. semi-short
    c. medium
    d. long

51. For a _____ style, clipper cutting is performed up to the occipital area and on the sides to the bottom of the crest.
    a. semi-short
    b. brush cut
    c. medium-length bi-level
    d. long

52. Razor cutting is especially suitable for all of the following *except* _____.
    a. thinning
    b. shortening
    c. feathering
    d. layers

53. The razor-over-comb technique is often used to taper nape areas or to _____.
    a. soften weight lines
    b. create design lines
    c. even the perimeter
    d. blend the perimeter

54. In the two-section method for razor haircutting, the hair is parted _____.
    a. from the ear across the crown
    b. from the forehead to the nape
    c. from the occipital ridge to the nape
    d. None of the answers are correct.

55. Replace dull razors _____.
    a. at the end of the day
    b. during a cut if necessary
    c. before each new client
    d. None of the answers are correct.

56. Thinning, slicing, and carving _____.
    a. are performed using clippers
    b. are only done with serrated shears
    c. are tapering techniques
    d. remove bulk

57. When shaving the _____ areas, hold the razor for a reverse backhand stroke.
    a. right side outline
    b. left side outline
    c. front hairline
    d. nape
    _____

58. A vertical subsection cut at a _____ projection can be cross-checked by parting off the subsections horizontally at 90 degrees.
    a. 0-degree
    b. 45-degree
    c. 90-degree
    d. 180-degree
    _____

59. When shaving an outline on _____ hair, first shave the front hairline.
    a. very short
    b. straight
    c. somewhat curly
    d. tightly curled
    _____

60. Clippers are used to facilitate _____ on a fade cut.
    a. tapering
    b. blending
    c. projection
    d. elevation
    _____

61. To create a crew cut, using a #1½ blade, cut with the grain, and angle the comb from the _____.
    a. left to the right
    b. right to the left
    c. crown to the front
    d. front to the crown
    _____

62. Use a changeable-blade straight razor to perform a _____.
    a. brush cut
    b. flat top
    c. head shave
    d. fade
    _____

63. When _____, remove excess hair using a balding clipper blade if available.
    a. shaving the head
    b. tapering the hair
    c. blending at the crown
    d. cross-checking
    _____

64. Shear-over-comb is the most popular technique for eyebrow trimming but a(n) _____ technique can be used as well.
    a. outliner-over-comb
    b. shear-over-comb
    c. freehand shear
    d. razor-over-fingers
    _____

65. Finger-styling produces a _____ look than brush styling.
    a. higher volume
    b. more textured
    c. smoother
    d. None of the answers are correct.
    _____

66. When _____ and the dryer are used to create wave patterns and direction in the hair, the technique is called blow waving.
    a. a diffuser
    b. a trimmer
    c. a comb or brush
    d. the fingers
    _____

67. One of the most popular types of _____ is on-the-scalp cornrows.
    a. braids
    b. finger styles
    c. locks
    d. None of the answers are correct.
    _____

68. To form a braid, place fingers close to the base and first cross the _____.
    a. center strand under the left strand
    b. left strand under the center strand
    c. right strand under the center strand
    d. center strand under the right strand
    _____

69. The comb is effective _____ hair locking.
    a. to maintain
    b. during the later stages of forming
    c. during the early stages of
    d. to remove
    _____

CHAPTER 16—MEN'S HAIR REPLACEMENT

Multiple Choice

1. Hair replacement systems have been worn for all of the
   following reasons *except* _____.
   a. as part of a ceremonial ritual
   b. to cover balding pates
   c. in conformance with fashion
   d. to keep the head warm   _____

2. In the eighteenth century, the word _____ was used to
   describe the front section of hair known as the foretop.
     a. toupee   c. side roll
     b. forelock   d. queue   _____

3. In current terminology, a hair replacement system is the
   term for _____.
   a. shaving your head and growing new hair
   b. artificial hair covering the head
   c. treating hair loss with drugs
   d. None of the answers are correct.   _____

4. Hair replacement options include all of the following
   except _____.
   a. treatment with minoxidil
   b. surgical hair transplantations
   c. scalp reduction
   d. a hair replacement system   _____

5. _____ hair is preferred over synthetic hair for a hair
   replacement system.
     a. Alpaca   c. Goat
     b. Horse   d. Human   _____

6. Hackling is the process _____.
   a. of performing an analysis before selecting a hair
      replacement system
   b. used to comb through the hair strands to
      separate them
   c. of a preliminary haircut
   d. None of the answers are correct.   _____

7. _____ hair tends to tangle most easily.
     a. Human   c. Animal
     b. Synthetic   d. Mixed   _____

8. Mixed-hair products, such as human hair blended with synthetic or animal hair, are often used in the manufacture of _____ wigs.
   - a. the highest performing
   - b. low-quality
   - c. low-cost
   - d. theatrical or fashion

   _____

9. Knotting refers to _____.
   - a. the way the hair is attached to the base of the hair system
   - b. the way the hair solution is attached to the head
   - c. the tendency of hair solutions to tangle easily
   - d. a cleaning technique for hair solutions

   _____

10. Root-tuning refers to _____.
   - a. the attachment of the hairs to the hair solution base
   - b. the way the hair solution is attached to the head
   - c. sorting the hair strands so that the cuticle points toward the hair ends
   - d. the density of the hairs in the hair solution

   _____

11. A new name for stock systems is _____.
   - a. faux-custom
   - b. pre-custom
   - c. template
   - d. sample

   _____

12. The supplies for hair solution services includes _____.
   - a. a blow-dryer
   - b. a razor
   - c. spirit gum
   - d. All answers are correct.

   _____

13. Before the preliminary hair cut, _____.
   - a. advise the client to shave his head
   - b. the client's hair should be allowed to grow fairly long
   - c. apply any chemical services
   - d. do not allow the client to wash his hair for a week

   _____

14. Measure from the client's nose to where the hair solution should begin using _____.
   - a. three fingers
   - b. four fingers
   - c. five times the client's eyebrow width
   - d. None of the answers are correct.

   _____

15. _____ using plastic wrap.
    a. Create a template for a custom hair solution
    b. Prepare the client's head
    c. Create the shape of the hair solution
    d. Protect the client's clothing   _____

16. Allow _____ to dry for 24 hours before sending to the manufacturer.
    a. a Styrofoam mold of the client's head
    b. the plastic wrap shape held with glue
    c. a plaster mold of the client's head
    d. the client's hair sample   _____

17. To customize a stock hair replacement system, first _____.
    a. comb the replacement
    b. arrange it over the canvas block
    c. shampoo and rinse thoroughly
    d. condition the replacement   _____

18. Apply two-sided tape in a V-shape on the front reinforced area of the foundation before applying a _____ system.
    a. reinforced   c. non-lace front
    b. unreinforced   d. lace front   _____

19. Attaching a hair replacement system to the head with _____ is called full head bonding.
    a. surgical methods   c. single-sided tape
    b. double-sided tape   d. an adhesive bonding agent   _____

20. A partial lace fill-in can be used for _____.
    a. a small degree of hair loss   c. 60 percent or greater hair loss
    b. curly hair only   d. complete hair loss   _____

21. After the first week, hair replacement systems should be cleaned _____.
    a. weekly   c. once a month
    b. every three to four weeks   d. every two months   _____

22. When permanent waving a hair replacement system, the system should be rinsed for _____.
    a. 1 minute   c. 10 to 15 minutes
    b. 5 minutes   d. 1 hour   _____

23. Do not recommend dark, opaque colors for _____.
    a. any age group   c. middle-aged men
    b. young men   d. elderly men   _____

24. A _____ percent solution of minoxidil applied twice
    daily has been shown to be moderately effective for
    about 50 percent of the men using it.
    a. .05   c. 10
    b. 2   d. 30   _____

25. Removing hair from _____ and transplanting it into
    the bald areas under a local anesthetic is called hair
    transplantation.
    a. another person   c. another part of
    b. normal areas of   the body
       the scalp   d. an animal   _____

CHAPTER 17—WOMEN'S HAIRCUTTING AND STYLING

Multiple Choice

1. Unisex salons _____.
   a. usually have a predominately male clientele
   b. maintain a fairly equal ratio of male to female clientele
   c. usually have a predominately female clientele
   d. do not provide as many services as barbershops   _____

2. All of the following are techniques for styling women's hair *except* _____.
   a. pin curls   c. hair wrapping
   b. thermal styling   d. dry setting   _____

3. Men's haircuts are more _____ than women's.
   a. rounded   c. angular
   b. soft   d. None of the answers are correct.   _____

4. Cross-checking involves checking for precision of _____.
   a. elevation   c. tapering
   b. line of blending   d. weight lines   _____

5. A blunt cut is _____.
   a. one length   c. another name for a crew cut for women
   b. formed using layers   d. graduated   _____

6. Cut with uniform minimal to moderate tension when creating a _____ cut.
   a. clipper   c. blunt
   b. graduated   d. layered   _____

7. For a blunt cut, comb the hair and part off into four sections from _____.
   a. front to center and center to back
   b. ear to ear and apex to nape
   c. front to nape and ear to ear
   d. right to left at the crown   _____

8. In a blunt cut, for the _____ design line, front guide length should be longer than back guide length.
   a. diagonal back   c. horizontal back
   b. vertical forward   d. diagonal forward   _____

9. The most common elevation for the _____ cut is 45 degrees
    a. blunt
    b. uniform
    c. graduated
    d. All of the answers are correct.   _____

10. _____ hair will graduate the most with a graduated cut.
    a. Coarse
    b. Curly
    c. Thick
    d. All answers are correct.   _____

11. In a uniform layered cut, all of the hair strands are cut _____ at a 90-degree projection.
    a. using a stationary guide
    b. to be even at the bottom
    c. at the same perimeter
    d. to the same length   _____

12. When creating uniform layers, establish a interior guide first, then set a guide at the _____.
    a. forehead
    b. crown
    c. perimeter
    d. nape   _____

13. When creating a uniform layered cut, long hair should be parted off into five sections: _____ panels.
    a. each side, one back, and two top
    b. top, two sides, and two back
    c. two top, two sides, and back
    d. None of the answers are correct.   _____

14. A _____ cut is achieved by cutting the hair at 180-degree elevation.
    a. blunt
    b. uniform layered
    c. graduated
    d. long layered   _____

15. When cutting curly hair, cutting _____ may encourage the hair to fall inward.
    a. just after the crest of the wave
    b. just before the crest of the wave
    c. just before the bottom of the trough
    d. just after the bottom of the trough   _____

16. With short natural cuts on _____ hair, the hair is tapered at the perimeter.
    a. straight
    b. wavy
    c. extremely curly
    d. somewhat curly   _____

17. Over-direction means that the _____.
    a. density of the hair is temporarily changed
    b. density of the hair is permanently changed
    c. hair is combed away from its natural fall position
    d. hair is shorter at the top than at the bottom _____

18. Point cutting is performed at the ends of the hair using the _____ at a steep shear angle in relation to the hair parting.
    a. tips of the shears
    b. still blade of the shears
    c. moving blade of the shears
    d. edge of a razor _____

19. Hair wrapping is a styling method that uses _____ as a form or tool.
    a. a block
    b. the fingers
    c. the client's head
    d. None of the answers are correct. _____

20. When performing hair molding, mousse and leave-in thermal styling spray are used after shampooing and _____.
    a. blow-drying
    b. air drying
    c. towel-blotting
    d. conditioning _____

21. When performing blow-dry styling, beginning in the nape area, insert the brush at the _____ of the section.
    a. top
    b. underside
    c. center
    d. base _____

22. When performing thermal waving, the projection of the hair from the scalp determines the _____ of the curl.
    a. size
    b. volume
    c. length
    d. None of the answers are correct. _____

23. The curl is _____.
    a. the foundation on which the barrel is placed
    b. the same as the volume
    c. the hair that is wrapped around the barrel
    d. between the scalp and first arc _____

24. A soft press removes _____ percent of the curl.
    a. 20 to 30
    b. 30 to 40
    c. 50 to 60
    d. 60 to 70 _____

25. When flat ironing, use a piece of misted tissue
    paper to _____.
    a. test the temperature   c. cool the client's hair
    b. wet the client's hair   d. All answers are correct.   _____

26. When performing flat iron pressing, divide the hair
    into _____ sections.
    a. two   c. four
    b. three   d. five   _____

CHAPTER 18—CHEMICAL TEXTURE SERVICES

Multiple Choice

1. Rods, _____, a waving lotion, and neutralizer are all used for permanent waving.
   - a. shampoo
   - b. conditioner
   - c. end wraps
   - d. relaxing cream
   _____

2. A soft-curl perm is also called a _____.
   - a. reformation curl
   - b. relaxer
   - c. soft wave
   - d. None of the answers are correct.
   _____

3. Relaxing cream, _____ or neutralizing shampoo, and conditioning product are all used for the relaxing process.
   - a. neutralizer
   - b. moisturizer
   - c. rods
   - d. end-wraps
   _____

4. The cuticle is the tough, outermost layer that _____.
   - a. protects the hair from damage
   - b. gives the hair its color
   - c. keeps the scalp warm
   - d. does not allow any chemicals to penetrate
   _____

5. Keratin is composed of _____ of polypeptide chains that make up the cortex of the hair.
   - a. hundreds
   - b. thousands
   - c. tens of thousands
   - d. millions
   _____

6. _____ types of cross-bonds hold together polypeptide chains.
   - a. Two
   - b. Three
   - c. Four
   - d. Five
   _____

7. Cystine is altered slightly to become _____ during chemical texture services.
   - a. keratin
   - b. cysteine
   - c. medulla
   - d. cortex
   _____

8. Neutralization reforms the _____ cross-bonds in the cortical layer.
   - a. hydrogen and cysteine
   - b. sulfur
   - c. hydrogen and sulfur
   - d. cystine
   _____

9. The rearranger _____ during a reformation curl.
   a. swells the cuticle
   b. inflates the medulla
   c. softens and breaks the internal hair structure
   d. re-forms hydrogen bonds _____

10. The waving lotion _____ during permanent waving.
    a. softens and breaks the internal hair structure
    b. forms a curl in the hair
    c. smoothes and shines the cuticle
    d. raises the medulla _____

11. In a permanent wave, waving lotion produces
    the _____ process.
    a. natural   c. physical
    b. biological   d. chemical _____

12. The neutralizer neutralizes any remaining waving
    lotion in the hair and re-bonds the newly arranged
    _____ bonds through a process called oxidation.
    a. hydrogen   c. sulfur
    b. cysteine   d. disulfide _____

13. _____ is the active ingredient in both the rearranger
    and the waving lotion.
    a. Cysteine
    b. Oxygen thioglycolate
    c. Ammonium thioglycolate
    d. Ammonium hydroxide _____

14. Lanthionization would most likely occur at
    a pH of _____.
    a. 3.0   c. 6.5
    b. 5.5   d. 11.0 _____

15. Lanthionization occurs as the _____ bonds are converted
    to lanthionine bonds.
    a. hydrogen   c. disulfide
    b. carbon   d. sulfur _____

16. When consulting about chemical texture services, discuss
    the client's _____.
    a. skin texture
    b. future vacation plans
    c. previous experience with chemical services
    d. weight _____

17. _____ should be recorded on the client record card.
    a. The price of the chemical service
    b. Information learned during the consultation
    c. The client's favorite color
    d. A receipt for the service   _____

18. Analyze the client's scalp _____.
    a. during the client consultation
    b. after washing his hair
    c. after applying the chemicals for perming or relaxing
    d. before proceeding with any chemical texture service   _____

19. The hair's porosity, _____, length, and direction of hair
    growth should be considered during hair analysis.
       a. texture   c. density
       b. elasticity   d. All answers are correct.   _____

20. Porous hair has a _____.
       a. raised cortex   c. flat cuticle layer
       b. flat cortex   d. raised cuticle layer   _____

21. Porosity is tested using hair from _____ different areas.
       a. two   c. four
       b. three   d. six   _____

22. When testing porosity, if the fingers _____, the hair is
    resistant.
       a. slide easily   c. do not slide easily
       b. form ruffles   d. feel oily   _____

23. The diameter of a single strand determines the hair _____.
       a. texture   c. porosity
       b. smoothness   d. density   _____

24. Coarse hair _____.
       a. typically requires the least processing
       b. typically requires the most processing
       c. tends to become discolored when permed
       d. can lead to a dry scalp   _____

25. Hair with _____ elasticity can stretch up to 50 percent
    of its original length without breaking.
       a. low   c. normal
       b. high   d. extremely high   _____

26. Sponginess is a sign of _____.
       a. porosity   c. resistance
       b. poor elasticity   d. low density   _____

27. Hair longer than 6" _____.
    a. is an ideal length for permanent waving
    b. may present problems with permanent waving
    c. requires shorter processing time
    d. requires longer processing time _____

28. Plastic rods are _____.
    a. only used for home processing
    b. the most commonly used
    c. not preferred by professional barbers
    d. all the same length _____

29. The _____ of perm rods usually vary from ⅛ to ¾ inches.
    a. diameters   c. circumferences
    b. lengths   d. None of the answers
                                  are correct. _____

30. Straight rods create a(n) _____ from one side of the hair parting to the other.
    a. half circle
    b. decreasing diameter
    c. increasing diameter
    d. consistently sized wave _____

31. A fishhook is a flaw that results in the _____.
    a. tip of the hair bending in a direction opposite to that of the rest of the curl
    b. curl forming only a semicircle
    c. part of the hair closest to the scalp remaining straight
    d. curl not maintaining its shape _____

32. The single flat wrap uses one paper placed _____ the hair parting being wrapped.
    a. under the top of   c. all around
    b. over the top of   d. under the bottom of _____

33. Perm wraps begin with sectioning the hair into panels that are further divided into _____.
    a. parts   c. subsections
    b. partings   d. base sections _____

34. A large diameter rod is used for _____.
    a. coarse thick hair
    b. fine hair with poor elasticity
    c. medium hair with average density
    d. medium hair with a smaller base section _____

35. In _____ placement, the hair is projected about 45 degrees beyond perpendicular to its base section and the rod is placed on the base section.
   a. off-base
   b. half off-base
   c. on-base
   d. None of the answers are correct.   _____

36. Half off-base placement results when wrapping the hair at an angle of _____ degrees to its base section.
   a. 0
   b. 45
   c. 90
   d. 180   _____

37. Wrapping with the natural direction of hair growth causes _____.
   a. the least amount of stress on the hair
   b. the highest volume curl
   c. the smallest curl
   d. hair breakage if too much waving lotion is used   _____

38. Spiral rodding can be accomplished in _____ ways.
   a. two
   b. three
   c. four
   d. five   _____

39. The pH of _____ generally falls within the range of 9.0 to 9.6.
   a. acid-balanced waves
   b. alkaline waving lotions
   c. true acid
   d. endothermic   _____

40. True acid waves use _____ as the primary reducing agent.
   a. glyceryl monothioglycolate
   b. ammonium thioglycolate
   c. hydrogen peroxide
   d. alkanolamines   _____

41. All acid-balanced waves have three product components: permanent waving solution, _____, and neutralizer.
   a. heat
   b. setting lotion
   c. activator
   d. None of the answers are correct.   _____

42. _____ waves use alkanolamines to replace ammonia.
   a. Exothermic
   b. GMTG
   c. Ammonia-free
   d. Acid-balanced   _____

43. Some permanent waving product packages contain
a pre wrap solution that is applied to the hair before
rodding; in most cases, this is a(n) _____.
   a. leave-in conditioner
   b. special shampoo
   c. thio relaxer
   d. acid-balanced solution
   _____

44. Mixing the contents of the activator tube with
a neutralizer will _____.
   a. make the activator more effective
   b. speed up processing time
   c. cause a violent chemical reaction that
      can cause injury
   d. make the solution too alkaline to be effective
   _____

45. A cold wave uses the _____ wrap method.
   a. lotion   c. post
   b. water or ice   d. lotion or water
   _____

46. _____ if the hair is not sufficiently processed after
10 minutes.
   a. Remove the solution and reschedule the client's
      appointment
   b. The solution should be reapplied
   c. Remove the solution to avoid damage
   d. Give the solution more time
   _____

47. Create preliminary test curls in _____ locations.
   a. two   c. four
   b. three   d. five
   _____

48. When a firm S curl is formed, _____.
   a. the hair still needs to be processed further
   b. the hair is over-processed
   c. curl development is complete
   d. the client's hair is too resistant for that
      particular solution
   _____

49. Hydrogen peroxide is the most common _____.
   a. neutralizer   c. leave-in conditioner
   b. activator   d. waving lotion
   _____

50. Most manufacturers recommend a _____ waiting period
before shampooing freshly permed hair.
   a. 4 to 6 hour   c. 24 to 48 hour
   b. 10 to 12 hour   d. one week
   _____

51. All the tools within a panel for a basic perm wrap are positioned in _____ on _____ bases.
    a. an alternating pattern; increasing size
    b. the same direction; decreasing size
    c. the same direction; equal-size
    d. a circular pattern; equal-size   _____

52. Because it _____, the curvature perm wrap is one of the best to use for men's styles.
    a. creates waves with small diameters
    b. produces a more natural-looking wave pattern
    c. has a limited amount of volume
    d. All of the answers are correct.   _____

53. If hair has been tinted or lightened before waving, _____.
    a. re-condition with a leave-in conditioner
    b. avoid waving for at least a week
    c. shampoo with an extra-mild shampoo
    d. avoid waving for a month or more   _____

54. Air conditioning may _____ of permanent waving solutions.
    a. slow down the action
    b. speed up the action
    c. ruin the results
    d. cause over-processing   _____

55. Always _____ applying waving and neutralizing solutions.
    a. perform a patch test right before
    b. use only one towel when
    c. protect the client's eyes when
    d. wear a mask when   _____

56. After examining a _____ and determining that the results are good, proceed with the perm, but do not re-perm the test curls.
    a. patch test   c. color sample
    b. test curl   d. texture sample   _____

57. When rinsing the waving solution, use _____ and a tepid water temperature, unless the manufacturer's directions state otherwise.
    a. firm water pressure   c. gentle water pressure
    b. a soaking basin   d. None of the answers
                                  are correct.   _____

58. A reformation curl, also known as a(n) _____ permanent, is a three-step process that is used to restructure very curly hair into looser and larger curls.
    a. true acid
    b. soft-curl
    c. cold wave
    d. ammonia-free _____

59. When performing a reformation curl, apply protective base cream _____.
    a. around the hairline
    b. above the ears
    c. only on the nape
    d. around the hairline and tops of the ears _____

60. Clients with extremely curly hair may prefer _____ services to straighten their hair.
    a. reformatting perming
    b. chemical hair relaxing
    c. chemical straightening
    d. physical relaxing _____

61. If there is an excessive buildup of dirty or styling products, _____.
    a. thio relaxers cannot be used
    b. perform a gentle shampoo service before using thio relaxers
    c. only hydroxide relaxers can be used after a normal shampoo service
    d. recommend that the client come back another day with cleaner hair _____

62. Thio relaxers have a pH above 10.0 and a higher concentration of _____ than permanent wave products.
    a. potassium
    b. hydrogen peroxide
    c. guanidine
    d. ATG _____

63. Sodium hydroxide is the _____.
    a. oldest chemical hair relaxer and is not commonly used today
    b. oldest and most commonly used chemical hair relaxer
    c. newest chemical hair relaxer but is not as effective as olderproducts
    d. newest chemical hair relaxer and is becoming very popular _____

64. Calcium hydroxide relaxers require the addition of a(n) _____.
    a. activator
    b. neutralizer
    c. lye solution
    d. alkaline solution _____

65. Ammonium sulfite has the _____ of all chemical
    hair-relaxing products.
    a. best effect on   c. lowest pH
       extremely curly hair   d. highest pH
    b. most lye   _____

66. Chemical blow-outs were used for many of the
    semi-straightened "Afro" styles of the _____.
    a. 1960s   c. 1980s
    b. 1970s   d. 1990s   _____

67. Applying relaxer to one small hair section is a _____ test.
    a. base   c. patch
    b. curl   d. relaxer   _____

68. Safety precautions for chemical hair relaxing
    include _____.
    a. using only one towel to avoid cross-contamination
    b. using a haircutting drape so that any excess hairs
       will slide off
    c. calling poison control in the event of accidental
       exposure to the client's eyes
    d. wearing gloves when applying relaxers   _____

69. Take _____ partings and apply base cream along each
    parting.
    a. ⅛"   c. ¾" to 1"
    b. ¼" to ½"   d. 2"   _____

70. During a retouch application, apply relaxer using _____.
    a. a brush   c. the back of a comb
    b. an applicator bottle   d. All answers are correct. _____

104

CHAPTER 19—HAIRCOLORING AND LIGHTENING

Multiple Choice

1. Early beard and mustache dyes were made from all of the following *except* _____.
   - a. silver nitrate
   - b. gold chloride
   - c. gum
   - d. indigo
   _____

2. The amount of elasticity and natural pigment in the _____ is an important consideration in determining haircoloring options and product selection.
   - a. cuticle
   - b. cortex
   - c. medulla
   - d. texture
   _____

3. Eumelanin gives _____ color to hair.
   - a. black and brown
   - b. red and yellow
   - c. black
   - d. brown
   _____

4. White hair is _____ percent gray.
   - a. 25
   - b. 75
   - c. 92
   - d. 100
   _____

5. _____ colors are red, yellow, and blue.
   - a. Bold
   - b. Primary
   - c. Secondary
   - d. Compound
   _____

6. _____-toned colors are predominantly red.
   - a. Cool
   - b. Fire
   - c. Fall
   - d. Warm
   _____

7. Green, violet, and orange are the _____ colors.
   - a. complex
   - b. rainbow
   - c. secondary
   - d. primary
   _____

8. Complementary pairs always consist of _____ colors.
   - a. three secondary
   - b. compound
   - c. two primary
   - d. all primary
   _____

9. The color wheel is a sequential arrangement of hues that makes _____ colors visible.
   - a. the relationship of colors
   - b. the shades of colors
   - c. only the primary
   - d. warm and cool
   _____

10. _____ colors are also called warm colors.
    a. Highlighting   c. Ash
    b. Light   d. Blue   _____

11. Level is the unit of measurement used to identify
    the _____ of a color.
    a. amount of blue tones c. degree of lightness
    b. amount of red tones   or darkness
                           d. saturation   _____

12. One is the darkest color on the _____ system.
    a. level   c. saturation
    b. hue   d. tonal   _____

13. Minimize _____ tones using blue base color.
    a. orange   c. violet
    b. red   d. yellow   _____

14. Hold a swatch up to the client's hair to determine
    the _____ of the hair.
    a. porosity   c. tone
    b. natural level   d. density   _____

15. Temporary color creates _____ color change.
    a. subtle   c. bold
    b. dynamic   d. permanent   _____

16. Permanent hair color _____.
    a. has an acidic pH   c. has the largest molecules
    b. fades gradually   d. has the smallest
                            molecules   _____

17. Temporary hair color _____.
    a. is acidic   c. causes a chemical change
    b. is slightly alkaline   d. lifts and deposits color _____

18. Concentrated rinses are mixed with hot water before
    application, processed for _____ minutes, and then
    rinsed.
    a. 1 to 3   c. 5 to 10
    b. 3 to 5   d. 15 to 20   _____

19. Direct dyes are also called _____.
    a. color rinses   c. demipermanent color
    b. semipermanent   d. haircolor mousses
       haircolor   _____

20. Color that lasts six to eight shampoos is _____.
    a. temporary   c. demipermanent
    b. semipermanent   d. permanent   _____

21. Demipermanent haircolor requires a(n) _____ before use.
    a. color rinse   c. low-volume developer
    b. special shampoo   or activator
                                  d. oxidizer   _____

22. Demipermanent colors are available in _____ form.
    a. gel   c. liquid
    b. cream   d. All answers are correct.   _____

23. Permanent hair colors do not contain _____.
    a. ammonia   c. peroxide
    b. oxidative tints   d. synthetic waxes   _____

24. The pH controls the _____ in a permanent hair color.
    a. final color result   c. processing time
    b. amount of lift   d. None of the answers
                                     are correct.   _____

25. _____ tints are also known as aniline derivative tints.
    a. Color-enhancing   c. Oxidation
    b. Direct   d. Toner   _____

26. Henna is a(n) _____ tint that is still used today.
    a. vegetable   c. metallic
    b. oxidation   d. mineral   _____

27. Metallic dyes _____.
    a. are also known as aniline derivative tints
    b. are very gentle on the hair
    c. are not recommended for use in the barbershop
    d. have a coating action and do not penetrate
       the cuticle   _____

28. A _____ is an oxidizing agent that supplies oxygen gas
    for the development of color molecules.
    a. developer   c. progressive
    b. neutralizer   d. tint   _____

29. A 10-volume solution corresponds to _____ percent
    H_2O_2 in water.
    a. 3   c. 9
    b. 6   d. 12   _____

30. Hydrogen peroxide safety precautions do not include _____.
    a. using clean implements
    b. avoiding contact with the skin especially at higher volumes
    c. not breathing in vapors from hydrogen peroxide mixed with other hair-color products
    d. only mixing hydrogen peroxide formulations in metal bowls

    _____

31. Avoid opening a plastic bottle of hydrogen peroxide _____.
    a. with a bulge
    b. that is older than one week
    c. that has been opened before
    d. with any damage to the label

    _____

32. Natural black hair will first be lightened to _____ during the lightening process.
    a. brown   c. gold
    b. red   d. pale yellow

    _____

33. Color oil lighteners add temporary color and _____ the hair as they lighten.
    a. highlight   c. lowlight
    b. curl   d. condition

    _____

34. Powder lighteners are also called _____ or quick lighteners.
    a. oil   c. neutral oil
    b. color oil   d. paste

    _____

35. Toners are available in _____ colors.
    a. primary   c. drab
    b. pale and delicate   d. ashy

    _____

36. Dye solvent diffuses and dissolves artificial pigment within the _____ layer.
    a. keratin   c. cuticle
    b. medulla   d. cortical

    _____

37. Both protein and non-protein fillers are manufactured in _____ form.
    a. gel   c. liquid
    b. cream   d. All answers are correct.

    _____

38. Most tint stains are removed from the skin using soap and water, but If that doesn't work, use _____.
    a. turpentine   c. a stain remover
    b. alcohol   d. hydrogen peroxide   _____

39. The patch test should be performed _____.
    a. behind the ear   c. on the neck
    b. inside the elbow   d. behind the ear or inside
                              the elbow   _____

40. When performing a strand test, place the parting _____.
    a. over a piece of plastic wrap
    b. over a piece of foil
    c. between your gloved fingers
    d. between your bare fingers   _____

41. A _____ is one of the materials needed for a strand test.
    a. towel   c. piece of plastic wrap
    b. fine-tooth comb   d. haircutting drape   _____

42. A soap cap is a combination of equal parts of a _____.
    a. prepared haircolor product and shampoo
    b. permanent wave and haircolor
    c. lightener and tint
    d. developer and oxidizer   _____

43. A _____ is the first step in a haircoloring service.
    a. patch test   c. thorough client
    b. scalp test   consultation
                           d. scalp analysis   _____

44. Pre-softening can be accomplished with a mixture of 1 ounce of _____ volume peroxide and 8 drops of 28-percent ammonia water.
    a. 10   c. 25
    b. 20   d. 30   _____

45. Lowlighting is also called _____.
    a. double-process   c. reverse highlighting
       coloring   d. a soap cap
    b. a strand test   _____

46. The foil technique involves _____ sections of hair to be placed on a piece of foil.
    a. slicing or weaving out c. cutting
    b. pinning   d. None of the answers
                              are correct.   _____

47. Temporary color rinses are used for all of the following reasons *except* to _____.
    a. bring out highlights
    b. temporarily restore faded hair color
    c. neutralize yellow tones in gray hair
    d. retouch permanent color   _____

48. When performing a temporary color rinse, a comb is used to _____.
    a. part the hair   c. straighten curly hair
    b. blend the color   d. None of the answers
                                 are correct.   _____

49. When using semipermanent color, hair will usually return to its natural color after _____ shampoos, provided a mild, non-stripping shampoo is used.
    a. 1 to 2   c. 6 to 8
    b. 4 to 6   d. 10 to 12   _____

50. Use a level 9 shade to color the hair of a client with a natural level of 6 who desires a level _____ shade.
    a. 6   c. 8
    b. 7   d. 9   _____

51. The first step in the procedure for semipermanent color is to _____.
    a. part the hair   c. put on gloves
    b. shampoo the hair   d. apply the color using
                                 a brush   _____

52. When using single-process haircolor, most color is formulated for use with _____ volume hydrogen peroxide.
    a. 5   c. 15
    b. 10   d. 20   _____

53. To _____, select one shade lighter than the natural color.
    a. remove tints from hair
    b. match the natural color of hair
    c. darken very light hair
    d. brighten, lighten, or cover gray   _____

54. For a virgin application, begin in the section where the hair is _____ or where there will be the most color change.
    a. thinnest   c. most resistant
    b. thickest   d. most porous   _____

55. _____ haircoloring begins with hair lightening.
    a. Double-process
    b. Single-process
    c. Retouch
    d. Lowlighting
    _____

56. Cream lightener generally is used for a _____.
    a. single-process application
    b. lightener retouch
    c. soap cap
    d. virgin application
    _____

57. _____ is indicated by gold pigments remaining in the hair after lightening.
    a. Damage
    b. Successful lightening
    c. Over-lightening
    d. Under-lightening
    _____

58. When lightening virgin hair, check lightening action by misting as for a strand test about 15 minutes before the completion of the time required. If the level is not light enough, _____.
    a. wait another 15 minutes
    b. wait another 30 minutes
    c. reapply the mixture
    d. None of the answers are correct.
    _____

59. Special-effects haircoloring includes _____.
    a. streaking
    b. frosting
    c. tipping
    d. All answers are correct.
    _____

60. The number of strands pulled through the cap determines the _____.
    a. degree of highlighting or lowlighting that is achieved throughout the hair
    b. time that the lighting solution should remain on the hair
    c. skill of the barber
    d. All of the answers are correct.
    _____

61. When performing the _____ over the entire head, the sequence of application should be lower crown, back, sides, top, and front.
    a. cap technique
    b. double-process color
    c. foil technique
    d. virgin application of single-process color
    _____

62. For _____ percent gray hair, permanent color should be applied at equal parts of the desired level and one level lighter.
    a. 10 to 15
    b. 30 to 50
    c. 50 to 70
    d. 75 to 90
    _____

63. Color fillers are dual-purpose haircoloring products that are able to create a color base and _____ in one application.
   a. de-frizz curly hair
   b. equalize excessive porosity
   c. straighten the hair
   d. curl the hair

   _____

64. When a barber encounters damaged hair, _____.
   a. he should suggest that the client avoid coloring
   b. he should suggest that the client avoid all chemical services
   c. the hair must be reconditioned before it can be tinted or lightened
   d. None of the answers are correct.

   _____

65. Lead dyes leave a _____ color, and those containing copper turn red.
   a. yellow
   b. gray
   c. purple
   d. blue

   _____

66. Pomades usually consist of harmless ingredients and are formulated specifically for _____.
   a. coloring mustaches and beards
   b. coloring the hair but not lighting it
   c. lightening the hair
   d. treating damaged hair

   _____

CHAPTER 20—NAILS AND MANICURING

Multiple Choice

1. Since 3000 BC, recorded history from _____ shows that nail care has been a part of human existence for a long time.
   - a. Egypt and China
   - b. Rome and Greece
   - c. Iraq and Persia
   - d. India and America

   _____

2. All of the following characteristics indicate good nail health except _____.
   - a. firmness
   - b. translucence
   - c. flexibility
   - d. opacity

   _____

3. Wavy ridges are a _____.
   - a. cause for extreme concern
   - b. permanent nail condition
   - c. sign of poor nail health
   - d. sign of good nail health

   _____

4. The nail bed is living skin that supports the _____ as it grows toward the free edge.
   - a. nail plate
   - b. matrix
   - c. lunula
   - d. cuticle

   _____

5. The _____ includes the lunula.
   - a. nail bed
   - b. epithelium
   - c. matrix
   - d. free edge

   _____

6. The seal between the _____ and the nail plate is formed by the cuticle.
   - a. nail fold
   - b. free edge
   - c. matrix
   - d. eponychium

   _____

7. The hyponychium is the slightly thickened layer of skin that lies between the _____.
   - a. cuticle and lunula
   - b. fingertip and the free edge
   - c. matrix and nail plate
   - d. eponychium and cuticle

   _____

8. Children's nails _____.
   - a. do not have a cuticle
   - b. have a larger lunula
   - c. grow most slowly
   - d. grow most rapidly

   _____

9. Bruised nails appear due to _____.
   - a. old age
   - b. fungal infection
   - c. an injury
   - d. malnutrition

   _____

10. Blue nails may indicate _____.
    a. stress
    b. systemic disorder
    c. malnutrition
    d. lack of hygiene
    _____

11. Paronychia is characterized by _____ of the nail plate.
    a. pus
    b. thickening
    c. brownish discoloration
    d. All answers are correct.
    _____

12. Ridges can be corrected with _____.
    a. nail filing
    b. careful buffing
    c. soaking the nails
    d. All of the answers
       are correct.
    _____

13. Hangnails can be improved by _____.
    a. softening the cuticles with oil
    b. cutting the nails very short
    c. allowing the nails to grow long
    d. careful buffing
    _____

14. Onychophagy is the medical term for nails that have
    been _____.
    a. weakened by disease
    b. infected by fungus
    c. damaged by blunt injury
    d. bitten enough to become
       deformed
    _____

15. Nail pterygium is an abnormal condition that occurs when
    skin is stretched by the nail plate as a result of _____.
    a. damage to the eponychium or hyponychium
    b. damage to the matrix
    c. biting the nails
    d. a genetic condition
    _____

16. In most cases, onychomadesis can be traced to a localized
    infection or minor injury to the _____.
    a. cuticle
    b. nail plate
    c. matrix
    d. free edge
    _____

17. Onychomycosis invades the _____.
    a. cuticle and spreads to the matrix
    b. nail folds
    c. eponychium
    d. free edge and spreads toward the root
    _____

18. The client's cushion should be covered with a _____ before
    each appointment.
    a. new neck strip
    b. clean towel
    c. heavy drape
    d. paper towel
    _____

19. A(n) _____ is an optional item used to shorten the length of time necessary for drying the client's nails.
    a. hair dryer
    b. lamp
    c. sanitized cabinet
    d. electric nail-dryer
    _____

20. Abrasive files are available in different grits; the lower the grit number, the _____.
    a. more gentle the action
    b. more aggressive its action
    c. smaller the file
    d. longer filing time is required
    _____

21. Hold the nail brush with the bristles _____.
    a. facing you
    b. turned down and away from you
    c. facing the ceiling
    d. facing the client
    _____

22. _____ are used to remove nail cosmetics from their containers.
    a. Disposable towels
    b. Cotton balls
    c. Plastic spatulas
    d. Terry cloth towels
    _____

23. Polish remover _____.
    a. contains organic solvents
    b. sometimes contains oil
    c. is used to dissolve and remove nail polish
    d. All answers are correct.
    _____

24. Use nail bleach to _____.
    a. remove yellow stains
    b. remove old polish
    c. lighten the color of polish
    d. None of the answers are correct.
    _____

25. Top coat is applied over colored polish to _____.
    a. darken the color
    b. lighten the color
    c. prevent chipping
    d. protect the fingers
    _____

26. Hand massage should end with _____.
    a. relaxation movement
    b. circular movement in the palm
    c. circular movement on the wrist
    d. circular movement on the back of the hands
    _____

27. When performing table set up, _____ 20 minutes before the first manicure.
    a. file your own nails
    b. turn on the lamp
    c. fill the disinfection container
    d. arrange items in the drawer
    _____

28. The pointed nail shape is suited to _____.
    a. male clients only
    b. clients who work with their hands
    c. hands that are on display
    d. thin hands with narrow nail beds   _____

29. When removing polish from a female client's hands, hold
    saturated cotton on the nail for approximately _____.
    a. 1 second   c. 10 seconds
    b. 3 seconds   d. 1 minute   _____

30. Hold an abrasive board at a 45-degree angle and file
    with an upward stroke to _____ the underside of the
    free edge.
    a. taper   c. bevel
    b. straighten   d. None of the answers
                                are correct.   _____

CHAPTER 21—STATE BOARD PREPARATION AND LICENSING LAWS

Multiple Choice

1. Self-doubt can lead to _____.
   a. overconfidence
   b. over-studying
   c. test anxiety
   d. None of the answers are correct.

   _____

2. Use your study skills _____.
   a. when studying for the practical exam
   b. when studying for the written exam
   c. by cramming the night before the test
   d. by reviewing at the last minute

   _____

3. Oral and/or written directions are _____.
   a. never given on a written test
   b. rarely provided for a test
   c. given at the beginning of a test
   d. None of the answers are correct.

   _____

4. When answering a(n) _____ question, first try to answer it in your head before reading the answers.
   a. multiple choice
   b. essay
   c. situational
   d. short answer

   _____

5. When answering a multiple choice question, if two possible answers are similar, _____.
   a. there is a mistake in the question
   b. they are both correct
   c. one of them is probably correct
   d. both answers must be wrong

   _____

6. When answering a essay question, make sure to write in a(n) _____ manner.
   a. complete
   b. accurate
   c. well-organized
   d. All answers are correct.

   _____

7. Situational questions _____.
   a. have only one question per scenario
   b. require a practical demonstration for the answer
   c. always require answers in paragraph form
   d. normally have more than one related question

   _____

8. The written exam covers _____.
   a. state barber board rules
   b. a demonstration of shaving
   c. a demonstration of a shampoo service
   d. the use of a model _____

9. Questions relating to barber laws may include _____.
   a. zoning rules   c. expected income
   b. the number of   d. tax laws
      board members _____

10. _____ is/are always covered on the practical exam.
    a. Continuing education c. Making appointments
       requirements   d. Chemical services
    b. Shampooing _____

11. On the practical exam, candidates must demonstrate
    competence with _____.
    a. a blow-dryer   c. shears
    b. outliners   d. curling irons _____

12. When practicing for practical exams, focus on all of the
    following except _____.
    a. requesting feedback
    b. timing yourself
    c. reading your state board rules
    d. studying different types of test questions _____

13. Which of the following statements is correct regarding
    the model you bring to the practical exam?
    a. You should practice on the model for several
       months.
    b. The model is provided by the state barbering board.
    c. The model makes travel arrangements for himself.
    d. Do not become too familiar or friendly
       with your model. _____

14. The practical exam _____.
    a. is offered in all states
    b. rules prohibit using your own tools
    c. requires that candidates wear a uniform
    d. may not be available in your own city _____

15. Avoid _____ the practical exam.
    a. wearing closed toe shoes for
    b. marking your kit bag with your name for
    c. arriving the night before
    d. disinfecting your tools before _____

16. Do not wear _____ for the exam.
    a. crocs   c. sandals
    b. clogs   d. All answers are correct.   _____

17. Before your exam, it is a good idea to _____.
    a. stay up late studying   c. get a good night's rest
    b. eat very lightly   d. celebrate with friends   _____

18. _____ are typically included in candidate booklets literature for the exam.
    a. Examination rules   c. Model names
    b. Examiner profiles   d. Study hints   _____

19. The state barber board conducts _____.
    a. disciplinary hearings   c. audits of barbershops
    b. public meetings daily   d. investigations into fraud   _____

20. The state barber board may discipline a licensee who is guilty of any of the following *except* _____.
    a. gross malpractice
    b. violation of the provisions of barber license law
    c. immoral behavior
    d. working at two salons   _____

CHAPTER 22—THE JOB SEARCH

Multiple Choice

1. The barbering job market _____.
   a. has a growing need for applicants
   b. is attracting many young people
   c. has been declining since the 1970s
   d. has been declining since the 1940s   _____

2. Prior to the _____, most average-sized towns had at least one barbershop.
   a. Vietnam War
   b. Beatles
   c. hippie generation of the 1960s
   d. All answers are correct.   _____

3. Forty years ago, _____.
   a. unisex salons were more popular than barbershops
   b. barbers also acted as surgeons
   c. most barber shops were franchise
   d. chain and franchise salons were virtually nonexistent   _____

4. In the early 1970s, _____ thought that "barbers and barbering are a thing of the past."
   a. the media
   b. everyone
   c. certain social and industry factions
   d. None of the answers are correct.   _____

5. Get a feeling for the atmosphere at area shops and salons _____.
   a. by interviewing their clients
   b. by interviewing their owners
   c. by visiting them
   d. All of the answers are correct.   _____

6. Keeping an open mind _____.
   a. will generate more income
   b. may hinder your relationships with clients
   c. can create more opportunities and probable successes
   d. is absolutely essential when becoming a barber   _____

7. Distributors and _____ sponsor student competitions.
   a. barber schools
   b. state governments
   c. state barbering boards
   d. None of the answers are correct.   _____

8. Office and classroom assistance may be provided by a(n) _____.
   a. teacher's aide
   c. receptionist
   b. apprentice barber
   d. fellow student
   _____

9. Strong work ethics are demonstrated by _____.
   a. a commitment to delivering quality service
   b. a belief that work is good
   c. a commitment to your employer
   d. All answers are correct.
   _____

10. The U.S. Internal Revenue Service (IRS) categorizes _____ as self-employed workers.
    a. independent contractors
    b. booth renters
    c. barbershop managers
    d. independent contractors and booth renters
    _____

11. As an employee, _____.
    a. your employer is responsible for withholding income tax
    b. you must work on a commission basis
    c. you must work on only a salary
    d. you do not get paid vacation
    _____

12. Independent contractors earning over $600 will receive a _____ for reporting taxes to the IRS.
    a. Form 1099-INC
    c. Form 1040-EZ
    b. Form 1099-MISC
    d. Form 1040-INC
    _____

13. A booth rental arrangement requires _____.
    a. that the shop owner report your wages to the IRS
    b. that the shop owner provides your supplies
    c. a contract with the shop owner
    d. All of the above.
    _____

14. Commission percentages depend on _____.
    a. your level of experience
    b. the number of clients the shop generates
    c. your agreement with the shop owner
    d. All answers are correct.
    _____

15. An employee with a salary of $10 per hour who works _____ hours per week could expect to earn $400 before taxes on $500 of service sales.
    a. 20
    c. 40
    b. 30
    d. 50
    _____

16. An independent contractor earning _____ percent commission only and working 40 hours can expect to earn $350 on $500 of service sales.
    a. 60
    b. 65
    c. 70
    d. 85 _____

17. A cover letter _____.
    a. serves as an introduction to an employer
    b. lists all of your educational experience
    c. lists all of your work experience
    d. includes pictures of your previous work _____

18. After you have passed your state board examinations, you _____.
    a. should contact the establishments where you are interested in working
    b. will be contacted by your new employer assigned by the state barber board
    c. should attempt to find a position teaching barbering
    d. are ready to set up your own barbershop _____

19. Which of the following questions would be appropriate to ask at an employment interview?
    a. Does the shop advertise regularly?
    b. When can I expect my first raise?
    c. When can I take a vacation?
    d. When do you see yourself retiring? _____

20. Employers are not permitted to ask _____.
    a. about drug use
    b. about citizenship status
    c. whether the applicant has been convicted of a crime
    d. whether the applicant smokes _____

CHAPTER 23—BARBERSHOP MANAGEMENT

Multiple Choice

1. Business ownership requires _____.
   a. financial management
   b. connections with local government
   c. a position on the state barbering board
   d. excellent barbering skills   _____

2. A _____ is a type of business organizational structure
   that may be considered for a barbershop.
   a. public company   c. cooperative
   b. non-profit   d. franchise   _____

3. A partnership involves _____.
   a. stockholders and managers
   b. the formation of a corporation
   c. a single owner
   d. two or more individuals sharing ownership   _____

4. A limited liability company can provide owners
   with _____.
   a. protection from acts or debts associated
      with the company
   b. extra investors who have no say over the company
   c. stock certificates
   d. None of the answers are correct.   _____

5. A(n) _____ arrangement is a form of compensation more
   often seen in chain or franchise salons.
   a. salary   c. salary-plus-commission
   b. commission   d. profit-sharing   _____

6. In a corporation, the _____ governs the management.
   a. owner   c. board of directors
   b. partners   d. federal regulators   _____

7. A(n) _____ owes the shop owner monthly rent.
   a. booth renter   c. independent contractor
   b. employee   d. partner   _____

8. The penalty for not reporting tips to an employer
   is equal to _____ percent of the social security and
   Medicare taxes due on those tips.
   a. 10   c. 50
   b. 30   d. 75   _____

9. When purchasing an existing shop, which question does the new owner not need to ask?
   a. Are there any defaults in the payment of debts?
   b. Is the mortgage, bill of sale, or lease transferable without any liens against it?
   c. Are there lease or current tenant obligations that have to be addressed?
   d. What type of work do the employees do? _____

10. In general, your target market should be reflected in the _____.
    a. number of employees
    b. shop location
    c. expected profits
    d. None of the answers are correct. _____

11. A lease protects the barbershop owner against _____.
    a. losing employees to rivals
    b. increases in taxation
    c. unexpected increases in rent
    d. loss of business _____

12. Under-capitalization is _____.
    a. the number one reason businesses fail
    b. easily remedied by bringing in partners
    c. not a major concern for a new barbershop
    d. only a concern for existing businesses _____

13. Two years of operating capital is not an unrealistic requirement _____.
    a. when opening a franchise
    b. when taking over an established business
    c. if there is no existing clientele
    d. if the owner is inexperienced _____

14. Local regulations do not include _____.
    a. local building codes
    b. zoning laws
    c. sales tax
    d. occupational or business licenses _____

15. An attractive, adequately furnished, and comfortable waiting area _____.
    a. is not important to most clients
    b. is only required when the rest of the shop has an unattractive appearance
    c. is prohibitively expensive to develop
    d. can be a promotional feature _____

16. Purchase insurance for _____.
    a. your employees to guard against loss of income
    b. in case you lose money from your business
    c. protection against fire and theft
    d. All of the answers are correct.   _____

17. Successful business operation requires an owner
    or manager who possesses all of the following
    except _____.
    a. diplomacy   c. at least 3 years
    b. good business sense   capital expenses
                                d. good judgement   _____

18. Expenses include all of the following *except* _____.
    a. rent   c. tax refunds
    b. utilities   d. salaries   _____

19. When the _____, a loss occurs.
    a. income is greater than the expenses
    b. expenses are greater than the income
    c. taxes are too high
    d. records are not kept properly   _____

20. All _____ should include the name and address of the
    client, and the date of each purchase or service.
    a. appointment records   c. client receipts
    b. consultations   d. service records   _____

21. When giving an employee positive feedback, follow all
    of the following guidelines *except* to _____.
    a. do so in a private area of the shop
    b. wait until his annual review
    c. give feedback right away
    d. be honest   _____

22. The cost of services is determined by _____.
    a. tax rates
    b. the salaries of the employees
    c. the type of clientele
    d. national averages   _____

23. During a typical workday, the barbershop telephone
    is used to _____.
    a. make appointments   c. order supplies
    b. seek new business   d. All answers are
                                   correct.   _____

24. When speaking on the phone, do *not* _____.
    a. worry about your   c. use a loud voice
       tone of voice   d. All answers are correct.
    b. hang up loudly   _____

25. Suggesting a temporary rinse _____.
    a. is a good way to sell hair coloring
    b. might be insulting to your client
    c. is not as profitable as permanent coloring
    d. None of the answers are correct.   _____

26. If a barber is not available for a client's request, _____.
    a. suggest other times he is available
    b. suggest another barber
    c. offer to call if there is a cancellation
    d. All answers are correct.   _____

PART II—Sample State Board Examinations

DIRECTIONS: Read each statement carefully. Choose the word or phrase that most correctly completes the meaning of the statement and write the corresponding letter in the blank provided.

SAMPLE STATE BOARD EXAMINATION TEST 1

1. The word *barber* is derived from the Latin word *barba,* meaning:
   a. to cut
   b. beard
   c. shave
   d. hairdresser _____

2. Barber-surgeons participated in the practice of:
   a. bloodletting
   b. tooth pulling
   c. surgery
   d. a, b, and c _____

3. In 1893, A. B. Moler established America's first barber:
   a. trade journal
   b. association
   c. school
   d. license _____

4. State barber boards are primarily interested in maintaining high standards of:
   a. appliances
   b. tools
   c. products
   d. competency _____

5. One key function of state barber boards is to protect the health, safety, and welfare of the:
   a. profession
   b. barbers
   c. public
   d. board members _____

6. Personality, personal hygiene, and attitude are all aspects of an individual's:
   a. grooming
   b. barbering skills
   c. professional image
   d. health _____

7. Proper behavior and business dealings with employers, clients, and coworkers are called:
   a. professional technique
   b. professional ethics
   c. career guidance
   d. behavioral characteristics _____

8. Pathogenic bacteria produce:
   a. health
   b. disease
   c. antitoxins
   d. beneficial effects _____

9. Pus-forming organisms that grow in clusters and cause abscesses, pustules, pimples, and boils are:
   a. streptococci bacteria
   b. staphylococci bacteria
   c. diplococci bacteria
   d. spirilla bacteria
   _____

10. Ringworm is caused by a/an:
    a. animal parasite
    b. poison ivy
    c. bacterial parasite
    d. plant parasite
    _____

11. Pediculosis is caused by:
    a. the itch mite
    b. the body or head louse
    c. scabies
    d. ringworm
    _____

12. The virus that causes AIDS is:
    a. HIB
    b. HIV
    c. ARC
    d. STD
    _____

13. The most likely manner in which HIV may be transmitted in the barbershop is by:
    a. shaking hands with an infected person
    b. blood-to-blood contact with an infected person
    c. using a soiled headrest
    d. using a sanitized comb
    _____

14. The removal of pathogens from tools and surfaces is known as:
    a. decontamination
    b. contamination
    c. sepsis
    d. cleaning
    _____

15. The process of thoroughly cleaning a tool or surface to its optimum level of decontamination in the barbershop is known as:
    a. sterilization
    b. sanitizer
    c. disinfectant
    d. disinfection or sanitation
    _____

16. State barber boards and health departments require only:
    a. sterilization procedures
    b. sanitation procedures
    c. disinfection procedures
    d. disinfection and sanitation procedures
    _____

17. A disinfectant that contains the properties of a bactericide, fungicide, pseudomonacide, virucide, and tuberculocide is considered to be a/an:
    a. minimal disinfectant
    b. hospital-level disinfectant
    c. deodorizer
    d. antiseptic
    _____

18. Antiseptics may be used on:
    a. the skin   c. dirty floors
    b. cutting implements   d. brushes and combs   _____

19. For effective sanitization, the minimum strength of
    a quats solution used to sanitize implements is:
    a. 10 percent   c. 1:1000
    b. 1:2000   d. 20 percent   _____

20. A wet sanitizer should contain:
    a. a disinfectant   c. an antiseptic solution
       solution   d. 2 percent formalin
    b. 30 percent alcohol   _____

21. The Occupational Safety and Health Administration
    (OSHA) regulates and enforces safety and health in the
    workplace by:
    a. setting safety   c. causing worker injury
       standards   d. importing products
    b. selling safe products   _____

22. Keep clean towels:
    a. near dirty towels   c. in a clean, closed cabinet
    b. in a clean, open   d. on a nearby shelf
       cabinet   _____

23. Barbers should wash their hands:
    a. in the morning   c. morning and afternoon
    b. when they get dirty   d. before and after serving
                                   each client   _____

24. Implements must be cleaned prior to immersion in
    a disinfectant solution to:
    a. avoid solution contamination
    b. comply with state board rules
    c. comply with sanitation procedures
    d. a, b, and c   _____

25. When a blood spill occurs, employ:
    a. a doctor   c. universal precautions
    b. safety precautions   d. decontamination   _____

26. Cream should be removed from jars with:
    a. the end of a used   c. a clean spatula
       towel   d. a comedone extractor
    b. the tips of fingers   _____

27. Hair or other waste materials on the floor of a barbershop should be:
    a. swept into a corner
    b. placed in closed container
    c. placed in a garbage can
    d. swept up at end of the day
    _____

28. Small nicks or cuts should be cleansed and treated with:
    a. a band-aid
    b. soap and water
    c. styptic powder
    d. a styptic pencil
    _____

29. The most desirable type of hair comb is made of:
    a. plastic
    b. metal
    c. bone
    d. hard rubber
    _____

30. The French type of haircutting shears:
    a. has no finger brace
    b. has one finger brace
    c. has two finger braces
    d. does not have a shank
    _____

31. When holding haircutting shears properly, the barber places the thumb in the thumb grip of the:
    a. shank
    b. still blade
    c. moving blade
    d. finger grip
    _____

32. Electric clippers are driven by a rotary motor, magnetic motor, or:
    a. circular motor
    b. pivot motor
    c. vibratory motor
    d. motor action
    _____

33. Headrest covers must be changed:
    a. for each client
    b. whenever they get soiled
    c. for every three clients
    d. for every other client
    _____

34. The size clipper blade that produces the shortest cut is:
    a. size 0
    b. size 0000
    c. size 000
    d. size 00
    _____

35. The first step in cleaning clippers and trimmers is to:
    a. brush off hair
    b. immerse blades in particles blade wash
    c. immerse blades in water
    d. spray with disinfectant
    _____

36. A straight razor is properly balanced when:
    a. the weight of the blade equals that of the tang
    b. the weight of the head equals that of the handle
    c. the weight of the blade does not equal that of the handle
    d. it does not pivot
    _____

37. The size of a razor is measured by the blade's.
   a. length
   b. thickness
   c. sharpness
   d. length and width
   _____

38. Honing and stropping are necessary for such implements as:
   a. haircutting shears
   b. thinning shears
   c. conventional straight razors
   d. hair clippers
   _____

39. The purpose of a hone is to:
   a. grind the razor's edge
   b. smooth the razor's edge
   c. polish the razor's edge
   d. align the razor's cutting teeth
   _____

40. The purpose of a strop is to:
   a. grind the razor's edge
   b. smooth the razor's edge
   c. polish the razor's edge
   d. impart a cutting edge to the razor
   _____

41. The shell or Russian shell strop is created from:
   a. the rump area of the horse
   b. cowhide
   c. synthetic materials
   d. canvas
   _____

42. The least acceptable method of removing loose hair after a haircut is the:
   a. small electric vacuum
   b. clean, folded towel
   c. unsanitized neck duster
   d. paper neck strip
   _____

43. An implement used to press out blackheads is a/an:
   a. tweezer
   b. comedone extractor
   c. electric hair vacuum
   d. electric latherizer
   _____

44. The basic units of structure and function in all living things are:
   a. nuclei
   b. cells
   c. centrosome
   d. living matter
   _____

45. The skull consists of eight cranial bones and:
   a. 8 facial bones
   b. 10 facial bones
   c. 12 facial bones
   d. 14 facial bones
   _____

46. The occipital bone forms the back and base of the:
   a. neck
   b. cranium
   c. upper jaw
   d. forehead
   _____

47. The more fixed attachment of a muscle to the bone is called the:
    a. origin
    b. insertion
    c. joint
    d. ligament
    _____

48. Muscle tissue may be stimulated by massage, electric current, and:
    a. heat and light rays
    b. nerve impulses and chemicals
    c. moist heat
    d. a, b, and c
    _____

49. The largest and most complex nerve tissue(s) in the body is/are the:
    a. lungs
    b. spleen
    c. brain
    d. heart
    _____

50. Nerves may be stimulated by high-frequency current, moist heat, and:
    a. chemicals
    b. light and heat rays
    c. massage
    d. a, b, and c
    _____

51. The main sources of blood to the head, face, and neck are supplied by the:
    a. jugular veins
    b. common carotid arteries
    c. arteries
    d. veins
    _____

52. The skin and its appendages make up the:
    a. integumentary system
    b. endocrine system
    c. circulatory system
    d. capillary system
    _____

53. The three types of matter are solids, liquids and:
    a. solutions
    b. mixtures
    c. gases
    d. compounds
    _____

54. The liquid that is considered to be a universal solvent is:
    a. alcohol
    b. peroxide
    c. bleach
    d. water
    _____

55. The best type of water to use in the barbershop is:
    a. distilled water
    b. mineral water
    c. soft water
    d. hard water
    _____

56. The pH of a solution measures its degree of:
    a. softness or hardness
    b. acidity or alkalinity
    c. heat or coldness
    d. neutrality
    _____

57. The pH range of hair and skin is:
    a. 3.5 to 4.5   c. 4.5 to 5.5
    b. 4.5 to 6.5   d. 5.5 to 6.5   _____

58. Acidic solutions will neutralize the effects of:
    a. alkaline solutions   c. heat or cold conditions
    b. salt solutions   d. stress on the hair   _____

59. A mixture of two or more substances that is made by
    dissolving a solid, liquid, or gaseous substance in another
    substance is known as a/an:
    a. solution   c. suspension
    b. ointment   d. powder   _____

60. Cosmetic preparations that will cause the contraction of
    skin tissues are:
    a. fresheners   c. facial toners
    b. astringents   d. a, b, and c   _____

61. The basic purpose of a cold cream is to:
    a. eradicate wrinkles   c. strengthen facial
    b. cleanse the skin   muscles
                            d. reduce fat cells   _____

62. Preparations that temporarily remove superfluous hair
    by dissolving it at the skin line are:
    a. depilatories   c. razors
    b. epilators   d. waxes   _____

63. Scalp lotions and ointments usually contain:
    a. surfactants   c. alcohol
    b. witch hazel   d. medicinal agents   _____

64. The primary ingredient in styptic powder or liquid is:
    a. talc   c. alcohol
    b. alum   d. witch hazel   _____

65. Witch hazel is a solution that acts as a/an:
    a. astringent   c. suspension
    b. emulsion   d. acid   _____

66. An electrical current flowing first in one direction and
    then in the opposite direction is called:
    a. direct current   c. alternating current
    b. tesla current   d. galvanic current   _____

67. Electric clippers and hair dryers are examples of barbering tools that use:
    a. alternating current
    b. converted current
    c. direct current
    d. rectified current
    _____

68. All electrical appliances used in the barbershop should be:
    a. barber board certified
    b. FDA certified
    c. UL certified
    d. OSHA certified
    _____

69. An applicator that directs electric current from the machine to the client's skin is a/an:
    a. conductor
    b. modality
    c. electrode
    d. massager
    _____

70. The high-frequency current commonly used in the barbershop is the:
    a. d'Arsonval current
    b. Oudin current
    c. sinusoidal current
    d. Tesla current
    _____

71. When using a Tesla high-frequency current on the face, what shape is the electrode used?
    a. flat
    b. rake-shaped
    c. oval
    d. square
    _____

72. Ultraviolet light produce:
    a. heat
    b. germicidal reactions
    c. chemical reactions
    d. b and c
    _____

73. Ultraviolet rays are usually applied:
    a. 12" to 16" from the skin
    b. 18" to 20" from the skin
    c. 20" to 24" from the skin
    d. 30" to 36" from the skin
    _____

74. The two main divisions of the skin are the epidermis and the:
    a. medulla
    b. dermis
    c. cuticle
    d. scarf skin
    _____

75. The outer protective layer of the skin is called the scarf skin or the:
    a. dermis
    b. adipose tissue
    c. epidermis
    d. subcutaneous tissue
    _____

76. The color of the skin is due to the amount of blood it contains and:
    a. keratin
    b. moisture
    c. fat
    d. melanin
    _____

77. The stratum germinativum is the innermost layer of the:
    a. dermis
    b. epidermis
    c. subcutaneous tissue
    d. corium
    _____

78. The dermis is also known as the corium, cutis, derma, and:
    a. cuticle
    b. false skin
    c. true skin
    d. fatty tissue
    _____

79. Subcutaneous tissue is also known as:
    a. muscle tissue
    b. soft tissue
    c. adipose tissue
    d. hard tissue
    _____

80. The sebaceous glands are duct glands that secrete:
    a. melanin
    b. sebum
    c. saliva
    d. perspiration
    _____

81. A structural change in the tissues caused by injury or disease is known as a:
    a. tumor
    b. lesion
    c. cyst
    d. fissure
    _____

82. Examples of primary lesions include all of the following *except:*
    a. bullas, cysts, macules
    b. vesicles, wheals
    c. papules, pustules, tubercles
    d. scars, fissures, keloids
    _____

83. Examples of secondary lesions include all of the following *except:*
    a. bullas, cysts, macules
    b. scales, scabs
    c. excoriations, crusts
    d. scars, fissures, keloids
    _____

84. A skin wart is known as a:
    a. keloid
    b. keratoma
    c. verruca
    d. nevus
    _____

85. The general term for an inflammatory condition of the skin is:
    a. trichology
    b. dermatology
    c. histology
    d. dermatitis
    _____

86. *Comedone* is the technical name for a:
    a. whitehead
    b. pimple
    c. blackhead
    d. patch of dry skin
    _____

87. Acne is a disorder of the:
    a. sweat glands
    b. oil glands
    c. intestinal glands
    d. stomach glands
    _____

88. An inflammatory skin disease that may be acute or chronic with dry or moist lesions is:
    a. eczema
    b. seborrhea
    c. psoriasis
    d. herpes simplex
    _____

89. A recurring viral infection that produces fever blisters or cold sores is:
    a. eczema
    b. herpes simplex
    c. psoriasis
    d. dermatitis venenata
    _____

90. The most common and least severe type of skin cancer is:
    a. squamous cell carcinoma
    b. malignant melanoma
    c. basal cell carcinoma
    d. melanoma
    _____

91. Hair is chiefly composed of a horny substance called:
    a. hemoglobin
    b. melanin
    c. keratin
    d. calcium
    _____

92. That portion of the hair found beneath the skin surface is called the:
    a. hair root
    b. hair bulb
    c. hair shaft
    d. hair papilla
    _____

93. A small, cone-shaped elevation at the base of the hair follicle is called the:
    a. dermal papilla
    b. hair bulb
    c. hair shaft
    d. hair follicle
    _____

94. Glands that secrete sebum to the hair and scalp are called:
    a. sudoriferous glands
    b. follicle glands
    c. sebaceous glands
    d. excretion glands
    _____

95. The three main layers of the hair shaft are the:
    a. cuticle, cortex, and medulla
    b. follicle, root, and bulb
    c. root, bulb, and dermal papilla
    d. follicle, root, and papilla
    _____

96. That portion of the hair that provides strength, elasticity, and natural color is the:
    a. medulla
    b. hair shaft
    c. cortex
    d. cuticle
    _____

97. Chains of joined amino acids are known as:
    a. amino chains
    b. end chains
    c. chemical chains
    d. polypeptide chains
    _____

98. Hair grows an average of:
    a. ¼" per month
    b. ½" per month
    c. ¾" per month
    d. 1" per month
    _____

99. The term used to indicate the number of individual hair strands per square inch of scalp area is:
    a. density
    b. porosity
    c. elasticity
    d. texture
    _____

100. The ability of the hair to absorb moisture determines its:
    a. level of density
    b. level of porosity
    c. level of elasticity
    d. variation in texture
    _____

101. Alopecia is the technical term for any abnormal type of:
    a. hair loss
    b. skin inflammation
    c. oil gland disorder
    d. sweat gland disorder
    _____

102. Common scalp disorders include dandruff, vegetable and animal parasitic infections, and:
    a. diplococcal infections
    b. streptococcal infections
    c. staphylococcal infections
    d. pediculosis infestations
    _____

103. Small, white scales appearing on the scalp and hair is a sign of:
    a. dermatitis
    b. eczema
    c. herpes simplex
    d. pityriasis
    _____

104. Ringworm of the scalp is the common name for:
    a. tinea
    b. tinea favosa
    c. tinea capitis
    d. tinea sycosis
    _____

105. All forms of tinea are:
    a. untreatable
    b. contagious
    c. non-contagious
    d. treatable by the barber
    _____

106. Scabies is:
    a. untreatable
    b. not contagious
    c. contagious infestation
    d. treatable by the barber
    _____

107. Inflammations of the follicle caused by bacteria or irritation may be signs of:
    a. folliculitis
    b. pseudofolliculitis barbae
    c. a or b
    d. neither a nor b
    _____

108. The main purpose of a shampoo is to:
     a. make hair easier to comb
     b. cleanse the hair and scalp
     c. treat alopecia areata
     d. soften the scalp   _____

109. Solutions that soften, swell, or expand the cuticle scales
     usually have a/an:
     a. acidic pH level   c. alkaline pH level
     b. neutral pH level   d. harsh pH level   _____

110. The portion of the shampoo molecule that attracts water
     and repels dirt is the:
     a. head   c. belly
     b. middle   d. tail   _____

111. The type of shampoo that is very effective in reducing
     dandruff is the:
     a. green soap shampoo
     b. therapeutic medicated shampoo
     c. liquid dry shampoo
     d. egg shampoo   _____

112. Rinses that are formulated to control minor dandruff
     and scalp conditions are:
     a. water rinses   c. medicated rinses
     b. bluing rinses   d. tonic rinses   _____

113. A cosmetic solution that can stimulate the scalp,
     correct a scalp condition, or be used as a grooming
     aid is a:
     a. conditioner   c. hair tonic
     b. styling spray   d. scalp ointment   _____

114. The purpose of a towel or neck strip between the drape
     and the client's skin is to:
     a. maintain sanitation standards
     b. conform to state barber laws
     c. prevent drape contact with client's skin
     d. a, b, and c   _____

115. The two methods employed by barbers to perform
     a shampoo service are the:
     a. upright and reclined methods
     b. inclined and reclined methods
     c. tub and shower methods
     d. backward and reclined methods   _____

116. Shampoo and scalp manipulations are performed with:
    - a. the cushions of the fingertips
    - b. the fingernails
    - c. rubber gloves
    - d. disposable gloves

    _____

117. Scalp massage should be performed with:
    - a. fast motion and no pressure
    - b. slow motion and no pressure
    - c. continuous, even motion and pressure
    - d. fast motion and heavy pressure

    _____

118. Barbers are qualified to perform treatments for all of the following except:
    - a. dry scalp
    - b. oily scalp and hair
    - c. dandruff
    - d. parasitic or staphylococcus conditions

    _____

119. Scalp massage is beneficial because it stimulates the:
    - a. salivary glands
    - b. blood circulation
    - c. pituitary gland
    - d. thyroid gland

    _____

120. Conditions that may prohibit a facial massage include the following except:
    - a. high blood pressure
    - b. severe skin lesions
    - c. skin inflammation
    - d. normal skin

    _____

121. A point on the skin where pressure or stimulation will cause contraction of the underlying muscle is a/an:
    - a. motor point
    - b. trigger point
    - c. sensory point
    - d. secretory point

    _____

122. Effleurage is used in massage for its:
    - a. stimulating effects
    - b. soothing and relaxing effects
    - c. heating effects
    - d. frictional effects

    _____

123. Facials performed in the barbershop are considered to be either:
    - a. preventive or corrective
    - b. corrective or medicinal
    - c. preventive or medicinal
    - d. corrective or therapeutic

    _____

124. The four skin types include dry, normal, combination, and:
    - a. sensitive
    - b. allergic
    - c. irritated
    - d. oily

    _____

125. When shaving a client, professional barbers use warm
     lather and a conventional:
     - a. disposable safety razor
     - b. straight razor
     - c. safety razor
     - d. electric razor

     _____

126. All of the following may cause ingrown hairs *except:*
     - a. excessively close shaving
     - b. shear cutting
     - c. excessive pressure
     - d. improper use of tweezers, razor, or trimmers

     _____

127. To achieve the best cutting stroke, the razor must glide
     over the surface at an angle:
     - a. against the grain of the hair
     - b. with the grain of the hair
     - c. across the grain of the hair
     - d. diagonal to the grain of the hair

     _____

128. When shaving, a gliding stroke directed toward the
     barber is used with the:
     - a. freehand stroke
     - b. backhand stroke
     - c. cutting stroke
     - d. reverse freehand stroke

     _____

129. Close shaving is the practice of shaving the beard
     during the second time over:
     - a. against the grain of the hair
     - b. with the grain of the hair
     - c. across the grain of the hair
     - d. diagonal to the grain of the hair

     _____

130. Facial shapes are determined by the position and
     prominence of the:
     - a. forehead
     - b. nose
     - c. chin
     - d. facial bones

     _____

131. A tapered haircut is usually longer in the crown and top
     areas and:
     - a. shorter at the nape
     - b. uniform at the nape
     - c. longer at the nape
     - d. neither a, b, or c

     _____

132. The removal of excess bulk from the hair is called:
     - a. slithering
     - b. dethickening
     - c. customizing
     - d. thinning

     _____

133. When using the shear-over-comb technique, the hair is placed in position for cutting by:
    a. combing through it
    b. holding hair between the fingers
    c. brushing through the hair
    d. rolling the comb out
    _____

134. The standard clipper cutting techniques are the:
    a. freehand and backhand
    b. clipper-over-comb and freehand
    c. freehand and underhand
    d. clipper-over-comb and backhand
    _____

135. The cutting method that can help make resistant hair textures more manageable is:
    a. clipper cutting   c. shear cutting
    b. razor cutting   d. hair singeing
    _____

136. Razor cutting requires that the hair be:
    a. chemically processed   c. clean and dry
    b. clean and damp   d. misted
    _____

137. Shaving the sides of the neck and across the nape with a razor is called a/an:
    a. extra service   c. neck shave
    b. outline shave   d. hairline shave
    _____

138. Hair replacement techniques include hair solutions (formerly known as hairpieces) and all of the following except:
    a. certain drugs   c. surgical hair
    b. chemical processes   transplantation
                                d. scalp reduction
    _____

139. Which of the following is not considered a type of surgical hair restoration:
    a. flap surgery   c. hair transplants
    b. knotting   d. scalp reduction
    _____

140. What is the first step in cleaning a ready-made wig?
    a. Brush to remove surface dirt
    b. Rinse the wig in cold water
    c. Pin the wig to a head mold
    d. Dip the wig into wig solution
    _____

141. The process used to chemically restructure straight hair into a different wave pattern is:
    a. permanent waving   c. reformation curls
    b. haircoloring   d. hair relaxing
    _____

142. A reformation curl is also known as all of the following *except* a:
    a. chemical blow-out
    b. Jheri curl
    c. soft-curl perm
    d. curl

143. The process used to rearrange over-curly hair into a straightened hair form is known as:
    a. a permanent wave
    b. a curl
    c. a reformation curl
    d. chemical hair relaxing

144. The two layers of the hair most affected by chemical texture services are the:
    a. cortex and medulla
    b. cortex and cuticle
    c. medulla and cuticle
    d. cortex and hair root

145. The partial or total removal of natural pigment or artificial color from the hair is called:
    a. hair lightening
    b. hair stripping
    c. haircoloring
    d. hair dying

146. The four classifications of haircoloring products include temporary and all of the following *except:*
    a. semipermanent
    b. permanent
    c. demipermanent
    d. temporary semipermanent

147. Temporary haircolor products are a type of:
    a. oxidation color
    b. penetrating color
    c. nonoxidation color
    d. self-penetrating color

148. Characteristics of permanent haircolor products include all of the following *except* that they:
    a. are mixed with hydrogen peroxide
    b. do not need retouch applications
    c. deposit and lift
    d. are penetrating tints

149. A patch test that results in redness or inflammation indicates the presence of a/an:
    a. immunity
    b. allergy
    c. blister
    d. verruca

150. The technical term applied to any deformity or disease of the nail is:
    a. onychosis
    b. melanonychia
    c. eponychium
    d. leukonychia

SAMPLE STATE BOARD EXAMINATION TEST 2

1. The word *barber* is derived from the Latin word *barba*, meaning:
   a. to cut
   b. beard
   c. shave
   d. hairdresser _____

2. Barber-surgeons participated in the practice of:
   a. bloodletting
   b. tooth pulling
   c. surgery
   d. a, b, and c _____

3. State barber boards are primarily interested in maintaining high standards of:
   a. appliances
   b. tools
   c. products
   d. competency _____

4. One key function of state barber boards is to protect the health, safety, and welfare of the:
   a. profession
   b. barbers
   c. public
   d. board members _____

5. Proper behavior and business dealings with employers, clients, and coworkers are called:
   a. professional ethics
   b. professional technique
   c. career guidance
   d. behavioral characteristics _____

6. Pathogenic bacteria produce:
   a. health
   b. disease
   c. antitoxins
   d. beneficial effects _____

7. Pus-forming organisms that grow in clusters and cause abscesses, pustules, pimples, and boils are:
   a. staphylococci bacteria
   b. streptococci bacteria
   c. diplococci bacteria
   d. spirilla bacteria _____

8. Pustules and boils contain:
   a. nonpathogenic bacteria
   b. pathogenic organisms
   c. sweat
   d. ringworm _____

9. During the active stage, bacteria:
   a. vegetate
   b. lie dormant
   c. grow and reproduce
   d. form spores _____

10. Ringworm is caused by a/an:
    a. animal parasite
    b. poison ivy
    c. bacterial parasite
    d. plant parasite _____

11. Pediculosis is caused by:
    a. the itch mite   c. scabies
    b. the body or head louse d. ringworm   _____

12. The virus that causes AIDS is:
    a. HIV   c. ARC
    b. HIB   d. STD   _____

13. The most likely manner in which HIV may be transmitted
    in the barbershop is by:
    a. shaking hands with an infected person
    b. blood-to-blood contact with an infected person
    c. using a soiled headrest
    d. using a sanitized comb   _____

14. The removal of pathogens from tools and surfaces is
    known as:
    a. decontamination   c. sepsis
    b. contamination   d. cleaning   _____

15. The process of thoroughly cleaning a tool or surface to
    its optimum level of decontamination in the barbershop
    is known as:
    a. sterilization   c. disinfectant
    b. sanitizer   d. disinfection or sanitation _____

16. State barber boards and health departments require only:
    a. sterilization procedures
    b. sanitation procedures
    c. disinfection procedures
    d. disinfection and sanitation procedures   _____

17. A disinfectant that contains the properties of a
    bactericide, fungicide, pseudomonacide, virucide, and
    tuberculocide is considered to be a/an:
    a. minimal disinfectant   c. deodorizer
    b. hospital-level   d. antiseptic
       disinfectant   _____

18. Antiseptics may be used on:
    a. the skin   c. dirty floors
    b. cutting implements   d. brushes and combs   _____

19. For effective sanitization, the minimum strength of
    a quat solution used to sanitize implements is:
    a. 10 percent   c. 1:1000
    b. 1:2000   d. 20 percent   _____

20. A wet sanitizer should contain:
    a. a disinfectant   c. an antiseptic solution
    b. 30 percent alcohol   d. 2 percent formalin
       solution

    _____

21. The Occupational Safety and Health Administration
    (OSHA) regulates and enforces safety and health in the
    workplace by:
    a. setting safety standards
    b. selling safe products
    c. causing worker injury
    d. importing products

    _____

22. Keep clean towels:
    a. near dirty towels   c. in a clean, closed cabinet
    b. in a clean, open   d. on a nearby shelf
       cabinet

    _____

23. Barbers should wash their hands:
    a. in the morning
    b. when they get dirty
    c. morning and afternoon
    d. before and after serving each client

    _____

24. Implements must be cleaned prior to immersion in a
    disinfectant solution to:
    a. avoid solution contamination
    b. comply with state board rules
    c. comply with sanitation procedures
    d. a, b, and c

    _____

25. When a blood spill occurs, employ:
    a. a doctor   c. universal precautions
    b. safety precautions   d. decontamination

    _____

26. Cream should be removed from jars with:
    a. the end of a used towel
    b. the tips of fingers
    c. a clean spatula
    d. a comedone extractor

    _____

27. Hair or other waste materials on the floor of a
    barbershop should be:
    a. swept into a corner
    b. placed in a closed container
    c. placed in a garbage can
    d. swept up at the end of the day

    _____

28. Small nicks or cuts should be cleansed and treated with:
    a. a band-aid
    b. soap and water
    c. styptic powder
    d. a styptic pencil _____

29. The most desirable type of hair comb is made of:
    a. plastic
    b. metal
    c. bone
    d. hard rubber _____

30. The French type of haircutting shears:
    a. has no finger brace
    b. has one finger brace
    c. has two finger braces
    d. does not have a shank _____

31. When holding haircutting shears properly, the barber places the thumb in the thumb grip of the:
    a. shank
    b. still blade
    c. moving blade
    d. finger grip _____

32. Electric clippers are driven by a rotary motor, magnetic motor, or:
    a. circular motor
    b. pivot motor
    c. vibratory motor
    d. motor action _____

33. Headrest covers must be changed:
    a. for each client
    b. whenever they get soiled
    c. for every three clients
    d. for every other client _____

34. The clipper blade size that leaves the hair the longest is:
    a. size 1
    b. size 2
    c. size 4
    d. size 3 _____

35. The first step in cleaning clippers and trimmers is to:
    a. brush off hair particles
    b. immerse blades in blade wash
    c. immerse blades in water
    d. spray with disinfectant _____

36. The grind of a razor refers to the shape of the:
    a. tang
    b. heel
    c. blade
    d. handle _____

37. The size of a razor is measured by the blade's:
    a. length
    b. thickness
    c. sharpness
    d. length and width _____

38. A crocus finish on the blade of a razor is also known as a:
    a. nickel-plated finish
    b. silver-plated finish
    c. plain steel finish
    d. polished-steel finish _____

39. The purpose of a hone is to:
    a. grind the razor's edge
    b. smooth the razor's edge
    c. polish the razor's edge
    d. align the razor's cutting teeth   _____

40. The purpose of a strop is to:
    a. grind the razor's edge
    b. smooth the razor's edge
    c. polish the razor's edge
    d. impart a cutting edge to the razor   _____

41. The shell or Russian shell strop is created from:
    a. the rump area of the horse
    b. cowhide
    c. synthetic materials
    d. canvas   _____

42. The direction used in razor stropping is:
    a. the same as that used in honing
    b. in a counterclockwise direction
    c. the reverse of that used in honing
    d. in a clockwise direction   _____

43. An implement used to press out blackheads is a/an:
    a. tweezer   c. electric hair vacuum
    b. comedone   d. electric latherizer
       extractor   _____

44. The least acceptable method of removing loose hair after a haircut is the:
    a. small electric vacuum
    b. clean towel, properly folded
    c. unsanitized neck duster
    d. paper neck strips   _____

45. The skull consists of eight cranial bones and:
    a. 8 facial bones   c. 12 facial bones
    b. 10 facial bones   d. 14 facial bones   _____

46. The occipital bone forms the back and base of the:
    a. neck   c. upper jaw
    b. cranium   d. forehead   _____

47. The less fixed attachment of a muscle to the bone is called the:
    a. origin   c. joint
    b. insertion   d. ligament   _____

48. Muscle tissue may be stimulated by massage, electric current, and:
    - a. heat and light rays
    - b. nerve impulses and chemicals
    - c. moist heat
    - d. a, b, and c
    _____

49. The parietal bones form the top and sides of the:
    - a. face
    - b. cranium
    - c. cheeks
    - d. neck
    _____

50. Nerves may be stimulated by high-frequency current, moist heat, and:
    - a. chemicals
    - b. light and heat rays
    - c. massage
    - d. a, b, and c
    _____

51. The main sources of blood to the head, face, and neck are supplied by the:
    - a. jugular veins
    - b. common carotid arteries
    - c. arteries
    - d. veins
    _____

52. The skin and its appendages make up the:
    - a. integumentary system
    - b. endocrine system
    - c. circulatory system
    - d. capillary system
    _____

53. Twelve pairs of cranial nerves branch out from the brain and reach parts of the:
    - a. arms and hands
    - b. legs and feet
    - c. abdomen and back
    - d. head, face, and neck
    _____

54. The liquid that is considered to be a universal solvent is:
    - a. alcohol
    - b. peroxide
    - c. bleach
    - d. water
    _____

55. The best type of water to use in the barbershop is:
    - a. distilled water
    - b. mineral water
    - c. soft water
    - d. hard water
    _____

56. The pH of a solution measures its degree of:
    - a. softness or hardness
    - b. acidity or alkalinity
    - c. heat or coldness
    - d. neutrality
    _____

57. The pH range of hair and skin is:
    - a. 3.5 to 4.5
    - b. 4.5 to 6.5
    - c. 4.5 to 5.5
    - d. 5.5 to 6.5
    _____

58. An example of a suspension is:
    - a. a quat solution
    - b. hair oil tonic
    - c. witch hazel
    - d. shampoo
    _____

59. A mixture of two or more substances that is made by dissolving a solid, liquid, or gaseous substance in another substance is known as a/an:
    a. solution
    b. ointment
    c. suspension
    d. powder
    _____

60. Cosmetic preparations that will cause the contraction of skin tissues are:
    a. fresheners
    b. astringents
    c. facial toners
    d. a, b, and c
    _____

61. The basic purpose of a cold cream is to:
    a. eradicate wrinkles
    b. cleanse the skin
    c. strengthen facial muscles
    d. reduce fat cells
    _____

62. Preparations that temporarily remove superfluous hair by dissolving it at the skin line are:
    a. depilatories
    b. epilators
    c. razors
    d. waxes
    _____

63. Scalp lotions and ointments usually contain:
    a. surfactants
    b. witch hazel
    c. alcohol
    d. medicinal agents
    _____

64. The primary ingredient in styptic powder or liquid is:
    a. talc
    b. alum
    c. alcohol
    d. witch hazel
    _____

65. Witch hazel is a solution that acts as a/an:
    a. astringent
    b. emulsion
    c. suspension
    d. acid
    _____

66. All electrical appliances used in the barbershop should be:
    a. barber board certified
    b. FDA certified
    c. UL certified
    d. OSHA certified

67. Electric clippers and hair dryers are examples of barbering tools that use:
    a. alternating current
    b. converted current
    c. direct current
    d. rectified current
    _____

68. The different types of currents used in facial and scalp treatments are called:
    a. units
    b. AC
    c. modalities
    d. DC
    _____

69. An applicator that directs electric current from the machine to the client's skin is a/an:
    a. conductor
    b. modality
    c. electrode
    d. massager
    _____

70. The high-frequency current commonly used in the barbershop is the:
    a. d'Arsonval current   c. sinusoidal current
    b. Oudin current   d. Tesla current   _____

71. When using a Tesla high-frequency current on the face, what shape is the electrode used?
    a. flat   c. oval
    b. rake-shaped   d. square   _____

72. Ultraviolet rays produce:
    a. heat   c. chemical reactions
    b. germicidal reactions   d. b and c   _____

73. Ultraviolet rays are also known as:
    a. actinic rays   c. tanning rays
    b. cold rays   d. a, b, and c   _____

74. The outer protective layer of the skin is called the scarf skin or the:
    a. dermis   c. epidermis
    b. adipose tissue   d. subcutaneous tissue   _____

75. The growth of the epidermis starts in the:
    a. stratum lucidum
    b. stratum germinativum
    c. stratum corneum
    d. stratum granulosum   _____

76. The color of the skin is due to the amount of blood it contains and:
    a. keratin   c. fat
    b. moisture   d. melanin   _____

77. The epidermis contains:
    a. blood vessels   c. adipose tissue
    b. small nerve endings   d. subcutaneous tissue   _____

78. The dermis is also known as the corium, cutis, derma, and:
    a. cuticle   c. true skin
    b. false skin   d. fatty tissue   _____

79. Subcutaneous tissue is also known as:
    a. muscle tissue   c. adipose tissue
    b. soft tissue   d. hard tissue   _____

80. The sebaceous glands are duct glands that secrete:
    a. melanin   c. saliva
    b. sebum   d. perspiration   _____

81. The duct of an oil gland empties into the:
    a. blood vessel   c. sweat pore
    b. hair follicle   d. hair papilla   _____

82. Examples of primary skin lesions include all of the
    following except:
    a. bullas, cysts, macules
    b. vesicles, wheals
    c. papules, pustules, tubercles
    d. scars, fissures, keloids   _____

83. Examples of secondary lesions include all of the
    following except:
    a. bullas, cysts, macules   c. excoriations, crusts
    b. scales, scabs   d. scars, fissures, keloids   _____

84. A skin wart is known as a:
    a. keloid   c. verruca
    b. keratoma   d. nevus   _____

85. The general term for an inflammatory condition of the
    skin is:
    a. trichology   c. histology
    b. dermatology   d. dermatitis   _____

86. *Milia* is the technical name for a:
    a. whitehead   c. blackhead
    b. pimple   d. patch of dry skin   _____

87. Acne is a disorder of the:
    a. sweat glands   c. intestinal glands
    b. oil glands   d. stomach glands   _____

88. An inflammatory skin disease that may be acute or
    chronic with dry or moist lesions is:
    a. eczema   c. psoriasis
    b. seborrhea   d. herpes simplex   _____

89. A recurring viral infection that produces fever blisters or
    cold sores is:
    a. eczema   c. psoriasis
    b. herpes simplex   d. dermatitis venenata   _____

90. The most common and least severe type of skin cancer is:
    a. squamous cell carcinoma
    b. malignant melanoma
    c. basal cell carcinoma
    d. melanoma   _____

91. Hair is chiefly composed of a horny substance called:
    a. hemoglobin   c. keratin
    b. melanin   d. calcium   _____

92. That portion of the hair that extends beyond the skin surface is called the:
    a. hair root   c. hair shaft
    b. hair bulb   d. hair papilla   _____

93. A small, cone-shaped elevation at the base of the hair follicle is called the:
    a. dermal papilla   c. hair shaft
    b. hair bulb   d. hair follicle   _____

94. Glands that excrete perspiration through the skin pores are called:
    a. sudoriferous glands   c. sebaceous glands
    b. follicle glands   d. excretion glands   _____

95. The three main layers of the hair shaft are the:
    a. cuticle, cortex, and medulla
    b. follicle, root, and bulb
    c. root, bulb, and dermal papilla
    d. follicle, root, and papilla   _____

96. That portion of the hair that provides strength, elasticity, and natural color is the:
    a. medulla   c. cortex
    b. hair shaft   d. cuticle   _____

97. Hair cells mature in the follicle through a process known as:
    a. cauterization   c. keratinization
    b. dissemination   d. propagation   _____

98. Hair grows an average of:
    a. ¼" per month   c. ¾" per month
    b. ½" per month   d. 1" per month   _____

99. The term used to indicate the number of individual hair strands per square inch of scalp area is:
    a. density   c. elasticity
    b. porosity   d. texture   _____

100. The ability of the hair to absorb moisture determines its:
    a. level of density   c. level of elasticity
    b. level of porosity   d. variation in
                                 texture   _____

101. *Alopecia* is the technical term for any abnormal type of:
    a. hair loss   c. oil gland disorder
    b. skin inflammation   d. sweat gland disorder   _____

102. Common scalp disorders include dandruff, vegetable and animal parasitic infections, and:
    a. diplococcal infections
    b. streptococcal infections
    c. staphylococcal infections
    d. pediculosis infestations   _____

103. Small, white scales appearing on the scalp and hair is a sign of:
    a. dermatitis   c. herpes simplex
    b. eczema   d. pityriasis   _____

104. Ringworm of the scalp is the common name for:
    a. tinea   c. tinea capitis
    b. tinea favosa   d. tinea sycosis   _____

105. All forms of tinea are:
    a. untreatable   c. non-contagious
    b. contagious   d. treatable by the barber   _____

106. Scabies is:
    a. untreatable   c. contagious infestation
    b. not contagious   d. treatable by the barber   _____

107. Inflammations of the follicle caused by bacteria or irritation may be signs of:
    a. folliculitis   c. a or b
    b. pseudofolliculitis   d. neither a nor b
       barbae   _____

108. The main purpose of a shampoo is to:
    a. make hair easier to comb
    b. cleanse the hair and scalp
    c. treat alopecia areata
    d. soften the scalp   _____

109. Solutions that harden, shrink, or constrict the cuticle scales usually have a/an:
    a. acidic pH level   c. alkaline pH level
    b. neutral pH level   d. harsh pH level   _____

110. The portion of the shampoo molecule that attracts dirt and repels water is the:
    a. head   c. belly
    b. middle   d. tail   _____

111. Hair loss characterized by the sudden falling out of hair in round patches is called:
    a. androgenic alopecia
    b. alopecia senilis
    c. alopecia areata
    d. alopecia syphilitica
    _____

112. Rinses that are formulated to control minor dandruff and scalp conditions are:
    a. water rinses
    b. bluing rinses
    c. medicated rinses
    d. tonic rinses
    _____

113. A cosmetic solution that can stimulate the scalp, correct a scalp condition, or be used as a grooming aid is a:
    a. hair tonic
    b. styling spray
    c. conditioner
    d. scalp ointment
    _____

114. The purpose of a towel or neck strip between the drape and the client's skin is to:
    a. maintain sanitation standards
    b. conform to state barber laws
    c. prevent drape contact with client's skin
    d. a, b, and c
    _____

115. The two methods employed by barbers to perform a shampoo service are the:
    a. upright and reclined methods
    b. inclined and reclined methods
    c. tub and shower methods
    d. backward and reclined methods
    _____

116. Shampoo and scalp manipulations are performed with:
    a. the cushions of the fingertips
    b. the fingernails
    c. rubber gloves
    d. disposable gloves
    _____

117. Scalp massage should be performed with:
    a. fast motion and no pressure
    b. slow motion and no pressure
    c. continuous, even motion and pressure
    d. fast motion and heavy pressure
    _____

118. Barbers are qualified to perform treatments for all of the following except:
    a. dry scalp
    b. oily scalp and hair
    c. dandruff
    d. parasitic or staphylococcus conditions
    _____

119. Cleansing the hair without soap and water can be
accomplished by using a/an:
    a. liquid dry shampoo   c. evaporating shampoo
    b. powder dry shampoo   d. a or b

    _____

120. Conditions that may prohibit a facial massage include
all of the following except:
    a. normal blood pressure   c. skin inflammation
    b. severe skin lesions   d. high blood pressure

    _____

121. A point on the skin where pressure or stimulation will
cause contraction of the underlying muscle is a:
    a. motor point   c. sensory point
    b. trigger point   d. secretory point

    _____

122. Effleurage is used in massage for its:
    a. stimulating effects   c. heating effects
    b. soothing and relaxing d. frictional effects
       effects

    _____

123. Facials performed in the barbershop are considered to
be either:
    a. preventive or corrective
    b. corrective or medicinal
    c. preventive or medicinal
    d. corrective or therapeutic

    _____

124. The four skin types include dry, normal, combination, and:
    a. sensitive   c. irritated
    b. allergic   d. oily

    _____

125. A scalp steam is not used to:
    a. relax and open the   c. soften the scalp
       pores   d. increase blood circulation
    b. close the pores

    _____

126. All of the following may cause ingrown hairs except:
    a. excessively close shaving
    b. shear cutting
    c. excessive pressure
    d. improper use of tweezers, razor, or trimmers

    _____

127. To achieve the best cutting stroke, the razor must glide
over the surface at an angle:
    a. with the grain of the hair
    b. against the grain of the hair
    c. across the grain of the hair
    d. diagonal to the grain of the hair

    _____

128. When shaving, a gliding stroke directed away from the barber is used with the:
    a. freehand stroke
    b. backhand stroke
    c. cutting stroke
    d. reverse freehand stroke
    _____

129. The once-over shave requires several strokes with each shaving movement:
    a. against the grain of the hair
    b. with the grain of the hair
    c. across the grain of the hair
    d. diagonal to the grain of the hair
    _____

130. Ingrown hairs are a common problem of:
    a. straight hair
    b. wavy hair
    c. coarse hair
    d. curly hair
    _____

131. A tapered haircut is longer in the crown and top areas and:
    a. shorter at the nape
    b. uniform at the nape
    c. longer at the nape
    d. neither a, b, or c
    _____

132. The removal of excess bulk from the hair is called:
    a. slithering
    b. dethickening
    c. customizing
    d. thinning
    _____

133. When using the shear-over-comb technique, the hair is placed in position for cutting by:
    a. combing through it
    b. holding hair between the fingers
    c. brushing through the hair
    d. rolling the comb out
    _____

134. The standard clipper cutting techniques are the:
    a. freehand and backhand
    b. clipper-over-comb and freehand
    c. freehand and underhand
    d. clipper-over-comb and backhand
    _____

135. The cutting method that can help make resistant hair textures more manageable is:
    a. razor cutting
    b. clipper cutting
    c. shear cutting
    d. hair singeing
    _____

136. Razor cutting requires that the hair be:
    a. chemically processed
    b. clean and damp
    c. clean and dry
    d. misted
    _____

137. Shaving the sides of the neck and across the nape with a razor is called a/an:
    a. extra service
    b. outline shave
    c. neck shave
    d. hairline shave
    _____

138. Hair replacement techniques include hair solutions (formerly known as toupees or hairpieces) and all of the following except:
    a. certain drugs
    b. chemical processes
    c. surgical hair transplantation
    d. scalp reduction
    _____

139. Which of the following is not considered a type of surgical hair restoration?
    a. flap surgery
    b. knotting
    c. hair transplants
    d. scalp reduction
    _____

140. What is the first step in cleaning a ready-made wig?
    a. Brush to remove surface dirt
    b. Rinse the wig in cold water
    c. Pin the wig to a head mold
    d. Dip the wig into wig solution
    _____

141. The process used to chemically restructure straight hair into a wave pattern is:
    a. permanent waving
    b. haircoloring
    c. reformation curls
    d. hair relaxing
    _____

142. A reformation curl is also known as all of the following except a:
    a. chemical blow-out
    b. Jheri curl
    c. soft-curl perm
    d. curl
    _____

143. The process used to rearrange over-curly hair into a straightened hair form is known as:
    a. a permanent wave
    b. a curl
    c. a reformation curl
    d. chemical hair relaxing
    _____

144. The two layers of the hair most affected by chemical texture services are the:
    a. cortex and medulla
    b. cortex and cuticle
    c. medulla and cuticle
    d. cortex and hair root
    _____

145. The partial or total removal of natural pigment or artificial color from the hair is called:
    a. hair lightening
    b. hair stripping
    c. haircoloring
    d. hair dying
    _____

146. The four classifications of haircoloring products include temporary and all of the following *except:*
    a. semipermanent   c. demipermanent
    b. permanent   d. temporary semipermanent _____

147. Temporary haircolor products are a type of:
    a. oxidation color   c. nonoxidation color
    b. penetrating color   d. self-penetrating color _____

148. Characteristics of permanent haircolor products include all of the following *except* that they:
    a. are mixed with hydrogen peroxide
    b. do not need retouch applications
    c. deposit and lift
    d. are penetrating tints _____

149. The technical term applied to any deformity or disease of the nail is:
    a. onychosis   c. eponychium
    b. melanonychia   d. leukonychia _____

150. Business operating expenses are also known as:
    a. overhead   c. credits
    b. accounts receivables   d. tax rebates _____

SAMPLE STATE BOARD EXAMINATION TEST 3

1. The first state to pass a barber license law was:
   - a. Minnesota
   - b. New York
   - c. Illinois
   - d. Ohio
   _____

2. Barber-surgeons participated in the practice of:
   - a. bloodletting
   - b. tooth pulling
   - c. surgery
   - d. a, b, and c
   _____

3. State barber boards are primarily interested in maintaining high standards of:
   - a. appliances
   - b. tools
   - c. products
   - d. competency
   _____

4. One key function of state barber boards is to protect the health, safety, and welfare of the:
   - a. profession
   - b. barbers
   - c. public
   - d. board members
   _____

5. Proper behavior and business dealings with employers, clients, and coworkers are called:
   - a. professional ethics
   - b. professional technique
   - c. career guidance
   - d. behavioral characteristics
   _____

6. Pathogenic bacteria produce:
   - a. health
   - b. disease
   - c. antitoxins
   - d. beneficial effects
   _____

7. Pus-forming organisms that grow in clusters and cause abscesses, pustules, pimples, and boils are:
   - a. staphylococci bacteria
   - b. streptococci bacteria
   - c. diplococci bacteria
   - d. spirilla bacteria
   _____

8. Pustules and boils contain:
   - a. nonpathogenic bacteria
   - b. pathogenic organisms
   - c. sweat
   - d. ringworm
   _____

9. The presence of pus is a sign of:
   - a. infection
   - b. impurities
   - c. immunity
   - d. healing
   _____

10. Ringworm is caused by a/an:
    - a. animal parasite
    - b. poison ivy
    - c. bacterial parasite
    - d. plant parasite
    _____

11. Pediculosis is caused by:
    a. the itch mite   c. scabies
    b. the body or head   d. ringworm
       louse   _____

12. The virus that causes AIDS is:
    a. HIV   c. ARC
    b. HIB   d. STD   _____

13. The most likely manner in which HIV may be transmitted
    in the barbershop is by:
    a. shaking hands with an infected person
    b. blood to blood contact with an infected person
    c. using a soiled headrest
    d. using a sanitized comb   _____

14. The removal of pathogens from tools and surfaces is
    known as:
    a. decontamination   c. sepsis
    b. contamination   d. cleaning   _____

15. The process of thoroughly cleaning a tool or surface to
    its optimum level of decontamination in the barbershop
    is known as:
    a. sterilization   c. disinfectant
    b. sanitizer   d. disinfection or sanitation   _____

16. State barber boards and health departments require only:
    a. sterilization procedures
    b. sanitation procedures
    c. disinfection procedures
    d. disinfection and sanitation procedures   _____

17. A disinfectant that contains the properties of a
    bactericide, fungicide, pseudomonacide, virucide, and
    tuberculocide is considered to be a/an:
    a. minimal disinfectant
    b. hospital-level disinfectant
    c. deodorizer
    d. antiseptic   _____

18. Antiseptics may be used on:
    a. the skin   c. dirty floors
    b. cutting implements   d. brushes and combs   _____

19. For effective sanitization, the minimum strength of a
    quat solution used to sanitize implements is:
    a. 10 percent   c. 1:1000
    b. 1:2000   d. 20 percent   _____

20. A wet sanitizer should contain:
    a. a disinfectant
    b. 30 percent alcohol solution
    c. an antiseptic solution
    d. 2 percent formalin

    _____

21. The Occupational Safety and Health Administration (OSHA) regulates and enforces safety and health in the workplace by:
    a. setting safety standards
    b. selling safe products
    c. causing worker injury
    d. importing products

    _____

22. Keep clean towels:
    a. near dirty towels
    b. in a clean, open cabinet
    c. in a clean, closed cabinet
    d. on a nearby shelf

    _____

23. Barbers should wash their hands:
    a. in the morning
    b. when they get dirty
    c. morning and afternoon
    d. before and after serving each client

    _____

24. Implements must be cleaned prior to immersion in a disinfectant solution to:
    a. avoid solution contamination
    b. comply with state board rules
    c. comply with sanitation procedures
    d. a, b, and c

    _____

25. When a blood spill occurs, employ:
    a. a doctor
    b. safety precautions
    c. universal precautions
    d. decontamination

    _____

26. Cream should be removed from jars with:
    a. the end of a used towel
    b. the tips of fingers
    c. a clean spatula
    d. a comedone extractor

    _____

27. Hair or other waste materials on the floor of a barbershop should be:
    a. swept into a corner
    b. placed in a closed container
    c. placed in a garbage can
    d. swept up at the end of the day

    _____

28. Small nicks or cuts should be cleansed and treated with:
    a. a band-aid   c. styptic powder
    b. soap and water   d. a styptic pencil   _____

29. The most desirable type of hair comb is made of:
    a. plastic   c. bone
    b. metal   d. hard rubber   _____

30. The French type of haircutting shears:
    a. has no finger brace   c. has two finger braces
    b. has one finger brace   d. does not have a shank   _____

31. When holding haircutting shears properly, the barber
    places the thumb in the thumb grip of the:
    a. shank   c. moving blade
    b. still blade   d. finger grip   _____

32. Electric clippers are driven by a rotary motor, magnetic
    motor, or:
    a. circular motor   c. vibratory motor
    b. pivot motor   d. motor action   _____

33. Headrest covers must be changed:
    a. for each client   c. for every three clients
    b. whenever they   d. for every other client
       get soiled   _____

34. The clipper blade size that leaves the hair the longest is:
    a. size 1   c. size 4
    b. size 2   d. size 3   _____

35. The first step in cleaning clippers and trimmers is to:
    a. brush off hair particles
    b. immerse blades in blade wash
    c. immerse blades in water
    d. spray with disinfectant   _____

36. The grind of a razor refers to the shape of the:
    a. tang   c. blade
    b. heel   d. handle   _____

37. The size of a razor is measured by the blade's:
    a. length   c. sharpness
    b. thickness   d. length and width   _____

38. A crocus finish on the blade of a razor is also known as a:
    a. nickel-plated finish   c. plain steel finish
    b. silver-plated finish   d. polished steel finish   _____

162

39. The purpose of a hone is to:
    a. grind the razor's edge
    b. smooth the razor's edge
    c. polish the razor's edge
    d. align the razor's cutting teeth   _____

40. The purpose of a strop is to:
    a. grind the razor's edge
    b. smooth the razor's edge
    c. polish the razor's edge
    d. impart a cutting edge to the razor   _____

41. The shell or Russian shell strop is created from:
    a. the rump area of the horse
    b. cowhide
    c. synthetic materials
    d. canvas   _____

42. The direction used in razor stropping is:
    a. the same as that used in honing
    b. in a counterclockwise direction
    c. the reverse of that used in honing
    d. in a clockwise direction   _____

43. Clipper blades are usually made of:
    a. tempered nickel   c. hard rubber
    b. chrome   d. carbon steel   _____

44. The least acceptable method of removing loose hair
    after a haircut is the:
    a. small electric vacuum
    b. clean towel, properly folded
    c. unsanitized neck duster
    d. paper neck strip   _____

45. The skull consists of eight cranial bones and:
    a. 8 facial bones   c. 12 facial bones
    b. 10 facial bones   d. 14 facial bones   _____

46. The occipital bone forms the back and base of the:
    a. neck   c. upper jaw
    b. cranium   d. forehead   _____

47. The less fixed attachment of a muscle to the bone is
    called the:
    a. origin   c. joint
    b. insertion   d. ligament   _____

48. Muscle tissue may be stimulated by massage, electric current, and:
    a. heat and light rays   c. moist heat
    b. nerve impulses and   d. a, b, and c
       chemicals

                            _____

49. The parietal bones form the top and sides of the:
    a. face   c. cheeks
    b. cranium   d. neck

                            _____

50. Nerves may be stimulated by high-frequency current, moist heat, and:
    a. chemicals   c. massage
    b. light and heat rays   d. a, b , and c

                            _____

51. The main sources of blood to the head, face, and neck are supplied by the:
    a. jugular veins   c. arteries
    b. common carotid   d. veins
       arteries

                            _____

52. The skin and its appendages make up the:
    a. integumentary system   c. circulatory system
    b. endocrine system   d. capillary system

                            _____

53. Twelve pairs of cranial nerves branch out from the brain and reach parts of the:
    a. arms and hands   c. abdomen and back
    b. legs and feet   d. head, face, and neck

                            _____

54. The liquid that is considered to be a universal solvent is:
    a. alcohol   c. bleach
    b. peroxide   d. water

                            _____

55. The best type of water to use in the barbershop is:
    a. distilled water   c. soft water
    b. mineral water   d. hard water

                            _____

56. The pH of a solution measures its degree of:
    a. softness or hardness   c. heat or coldness
    b. acidity or alkalinity   d. neutrality

                            _____

57. The pH range of hair and skin is:
    a. 3.5 to 4.5   c. 4.5 to 5.5
    b. 4.5 to 6.5   d. 5.5 to 6.5

                            _____

58. An example of a suspension is:
    a. a quat solution   c. witch hazel
    b. hair oil tonic   d. shampoo

                            _____

59. A mixture of two or more substances that is made by dissolving a solid, liquid, or gaseous substance in another substance is known as a/an:
    a. solution
    b. ointment
    c. suspension
    d. powder
    _____

60. Cosmetic preparations that will cause the contraction of skin tissues are:
    a. fresheners
    b. astringents
    c. facial toners
    d. a, b, and c
    _____

61. The basic purpose of a cold cream is to:
    a. eradicate wrinkles
    b. cleanse the skin
    c. strengthen facial muscles
    d. reduce fat cells
    _____

62. Preparations that temporarily remove superfluous hair by dissolving it at the skin line are:
    a. depilatories
    b. epilators
    c. razors
    d. waxes
    _____

63. Scalp lotions and ointments usually contain:
    a. surfactants
    b. witch hazel
    c. alcohol
    d. medicinal agents
    _____

64. The primary ingredient in styptic powder or liquid is:
    a. talc
    b. alum
    c. alcohol
    d. witch hazel
    _____

65. Witch hazel is a solution that acts as a/an:
    a. astringent
    b. emulsion
    c. suspension
    d. acid
    _____

66. All electrical appliances used in the barbershop should be:
    a. barber board certified
    b. FDA certified
    c. UL certified
    d. OSHA certified
    _____

67. Electric clippers and hair dryers are examples of barbering tools that use:
    a. alternating current
    b. converted current
    c. direct current
    d. rectified current
    _____

68. The different types of currents used in facial and scalp treatments are called:
    a. units
    b. AC
    c. modalities
    d. DC
    _____

69. An applicator that directs electric current from the machine to the client's skin is a/an:
    a. conductor
    b. modality
    c. electrode
    d. massager _____

70. The high-frequency current commonly used in the barbershop is the:
    a. d'Arsonval current
    b. Oudin current
    c. sinusoidal current
    d. Tesla current _____

71. When using a Tesla high-frequency current on the face, what shape is the electrode used?
    a. flat
    b. rake-shaped
    c. oval
    d. square _____

72. Ultraviolet light produce:
    a. heat
    b. germicidal reactions
    c. chemical reactions
    d. b and c _____

73. Ultraviolet rays are also known as:
    a. actinic rays
    b. cold rays
    c. tanning rays
    d. a, b, and c _____

74. The outer protective layer of the skin is called the scarf skin or the:
    a. dermis
    b. adipose tissue
    c. epidermis
    d. subcutaneous tissue _____

75. The layer of the epidermis that is continually shed is the:
    a. stratum lucidum
    b. stratum germinativum
    c. stratum corneum
    d. stratum granulosum _____

76. The color of the skin is due to the amount of blood it contains and:
    a. keratin
    b. moisture
    c. fat
    d. melanin _____

77. The epidermis contains:
    a. blood vessels
    b. small nerve endings
    c. adipose tissue
    d. subcutaneous tissue _____

78. The dermis is also known as the corium, cutis, derma, and:
    a. cuticle
    b. false skin
    c. true skin
    d. fatty tissue _____

79. Subcutaneous tissue is also known as:
    a. muscle tissue   c. adipose tissue
    b. soft tissue   d. hard tissue   _____

80. The sebaceous glands are duct glands that secrete:
    a. melanin   c. saliva
    b. sebum   d. perspiration   _____

81. The duct of an oil gland empties into the:
    a. blood vessel   c. sweat pore
    b. hair follicle   d. hair papilla   _____

82. Examples of primary skin lesions include all of the
    following *except:*
    a. bullas, cysts, macules
    b. vesicles, wheals
    c. papules, pustules, tubercles
    d. scars, fissures, keloids   _____

83. Examples of secondary lesions include all of the
    following *except:*
    a. bullas, cysts, macules   c. excoriations, crusts
    b. scales, scabs   d. scars, fissures, keloids   _____

84. A skin wart is known as a:
    a. keloid   c. verruca
    b. keratoma   d. nevus   _____

85. The general term for an inflammatory condition of the
    skin is:
    a. trichology   c. histology
    b. dermatology   d. dermatitis   _____

86. *Milia* is the technical name for a:
    a. whitehead   c. blackhead
    b. pimple   d. patch of dry skin   _____

87. Acne is a disorder of the:
    a. sweat glands   c. intestinal glands
    b. oil glands   d. stomach glands   _____

88. A chronic, inflammatory skin disease with dry red
    patches and coarse silvery scales is:
    a. eczema   c. psoriasis
    b. herpes simplex   d. dermatitis venenata _____

89. A recurring viral infection that produces fever blisters or cold sores is:
    a. eczema
    b. herpes simplex
    c. psoriasis
    d. dermatitis venenata
    _____

90. The most common and least severe type of skin cancer is:
    a. squamous cell carcinoma
    b. malignant melanoma
    c. basal cell carcinoma
    d. melanoma
    _____

91. Hair is chiefly composed of a horny substance called:
    a. hemoglobin
    b. melanin
    c. keratin
    d. calcium
    _____

92. That portion of the hair that extends beyond the skin surface is called the:
    a. hair root
    b. hair bulb
    c. hair shaft
    d. hair papilla
    _____

93. A small, cone-shaped elevation at the base of the hair follicle is called the:
    a. dermal papilla
    b. hair bulb
    c. hair shaft
    d. hair follicle
    _____

94. Glands that excrete perspiration through the skin pores are called:
    a. sudoriferous glands
    b. follicle glands
    c. sebaceous glands
    d. excretion glands
    _____

95. The three main layers of the hair shaft are the:
    a. cuticle, cortex, and medulla
    b. follicle, root, and bulb
    c. root, bulb, and dermal papilla
    d. follicle, root, and papilla
    _____

96. That portion of the hair that provides strength, elasticity, and natural color is the:
    a. medulla
    b. hair shaft
    c. cortex
    d. cuticle
    _____

97. Hair cells mature in the follicle through a process known as:
    a. cauterization
    b. dissemination
    c. keratinization
    d. propagation
    _____

98. Hair grows an average of:
    a. ¼" per month
    b. ½" per month
    c. ¾" per month
    d. 1" per month
    _____

99. The term used to indicate the number of individual hair strands per square inch of scalp area is:
    a. density
    c. elasticity
    b. porosity
    d. texture
    _____

100. The ability of the hair to absorb moisture determines its:
    a. level of density
    c. level of elasticity
    b. level of porosity
    d. variation in texture
    _____

101. *Alopecia* is the technical term for any abnormal type of:
    a. hair loss
    c. oil gland disorder
    b. skin inflammation
    d. sweat gland disorder
    _____

102. Common scalp disorders include dandruff, vegetable and animal parasitic infections, and:
    a. diplococcal infections
    b. streptococcal infections
    c. staphylococcal infections
    d. pediculosis infestations
    _____

103. Small, white scales appearing on the scalp and hair is a sign of:
    a. dermatitis
    c. herpes simplex
    b. eczema
    d. pityriasis
    _____

104. Ringworm of the scalp is the common name for:
    a. tinea
    c. tinea capitis
    b. tinea favosa
    d. tinea sycosis
    _____

105. All forms of tinea are:
    a. untreatable
    c. non-contagious
    b. contagious
    d. treatable by the barber
    _____

106. Scabies is:
    a. untreatable
    c. contagious infestation
    b. not contagious
    d. treatable by the barber
    _____

107. Inflammations of the follicle caused by bacteria or irritation may be signs of:
    a. folliculitis
    c. a or b
    b. pseudofolliculitis barbae
    d. neither a nor b
    _____

108. The main purpose of a shampoo is to:
    a. make hair easier to comb
    b. cleanse the hair and scalp
    c. treat alopecia areata
    d. soften the scalp
    _____

109. Solutions that harden, shrink, or constrict the cuticle scales usually have a/an:
    a. acidic pH level
    b. neutral pH level
    c. alkaline pH level
    d. harsh pH level
    _____

110. The portion of the shampoo molecule that attracts dirt and repels water is the:
    a. head
    b. middle
    c. belly
    d. tail
    _____

111. Hair loss characterized by the sudden falling out of hair in round patches is called:
    a. androgenic alopecia
    b. alopecia senilis
    c. alopecia areata
    d. alopecia syphilitica
    _____

112. Rinses that are formulated to control minor dandruff and scalp conditions are:
    a. water rinses
    b. bluing rinses
    c. medicated rinses
    d. tonic rinses
    _____

113. A cosmetic solution that can stimulate the scalp, correct a scalp condition, or be used as a grooming aid is a:
    a. hair tonic
    b. styling spray
    c. conditioner
    d. scalp ointment
    _____

114. The purpose of a towel or neck strip between the drape and the client's skin is to:
    a. maintain sanitation standards
    b. conform to state barber laws
    c. prevent drape contact with client's skin
    d. a, b, and c
    _____

115. The two methods employed by barbers to perform a shampoo service are the:
    a. upright and reclined methods
    b. inclined and reclined methods
    c. tub and shower methods
    d. backward and reclined methods
    _____

116. Shampoo and scalp manipulations are performed with:
    a. the cushions of the fingertips
    b. the fingernails
    c. rubber gloves
    d. disposable gloves
    _____

117. Scalp massage should be performed with:
     a. fast motion and no pressure
     b. slow motion and no pressure
     c. continuous, even motion and pressure
     d. fast motion and heavy pressure
     _____

118. Barbers are qualified to perform treatments for all of
     the following *except*:
     a. dry scalp
     b. oily scalp and hair
     c. dandruff
     d. parasitic or staphylococcus conditions
     _____

119. Cleansing the hair without soap and water can be
     accomplished by using a/an:
     a. liquid dry shampoo   c. evaporating shampoo
     b. powder dry shampoo   d. a or b
     _____

120. Conditions that may prohibit a facial massage include
     all of the following *except*:
     a. normal blood   c. skin inflammation
        pressure   d. high blood pressure
     b. severe skin lesions
     _____

121. A point on the skin where pressure or stimulation will
     cause contraction of the underlying muscle is a/an:
     a. motor point   c. sensory point
     b. trigger point   d. secretory point
     _____

122. Pétrissage is the type of massage movement involving:
     a. friction   c. kneading or pinching
     b. percussion   d. tapotement
     _____

123. Effleurage is used in massage for its:
     a. stimulating effects   c. heating effects
     b. soothing and   d. frictional effects
        relaxing effects
     _____

124. The four skin types include dry, normal, oily, and:
     a. sensitive   c. irritated
     b. allergic   d. combination
     _____

125. A scalp steam *is not* used to:
     a. relax and open   c. soften the scalp
        the pores   d. increase blood circulation
     b. close the pores
     _____

126. All of the following may cause ingrown hairs *except*:
     a. excessively close shaving
     b. shear cutting
     c. excessive pressure
     d. improper use of tweezers, razor, or trimmers _____

127. To achieve the best cutting stroke, the razor must glide
     over the surface at an angle:
     a. with the grain of the hair
     b. against the grain of the hair
     c. across the grain of the hair
     d. diagonal to the grain of the hair _____

128. When shaving, a gliding stroke directed away from the
     barber is used with the:
     a. freehand stroke   c. cutting stroke
     b. backhand stroke   d. reverse freehand stroke _____

129. The once-over shave requires several strokes with each
     shaving movement:
     a. against the grain of the hair
     b. with the grain of the hair
     c. across the grain of the hair
     d. diagonal to the grain of the hair _____

130. Ingrown hairs are a common problem of:
     a. straight hair   c. coarse hair
     b. wavy hair   d. curly hair _____

131. A tapered haircut is longer in the crown and top areas and:
     a. shorter at the nape   c. longer at the nape
     b. uniform at the nape   d. neither a, b, or c _____

132. The removal of excess bulk from the hair is called:
     a. slithering   c. customizing
     b. dethickening   d. thinning _____

133. When using the shear-over-comb technique, the hair is
     placed in position for cutting by:
     a. combing through it   c. brushing through the hair
     b. holding it between   d. rolling the comb out _____
        the fingers

134. The standard clipper cutting techniques are the:
     a. freehand and backhand
     b. clipper-over-comb and freehand
     c. freehand and underhand
     d. clipper-over-comb and backhand _____

172

135. The type of cutting method that can help make resistant hair textures more manageable is:
    a. razor cutting
    b. clipper cutting
    c. shear cutting
    d. hair singeing
    _____

136. Razor cutting requires that the hair be:
    a. chemically processed
    b. clean and damp
    c. clean and dry
    d. misted
    _____

137. Shaving the sides of the neck and across the nape with a razor is called a/an:
    a. extra service
    b. outline shave
    c. neck shave
    d. hairline shave
    _____

138. Hair replacement techniques include hair solutions (formerly known as toupees or hairpieces) and all of the following *except*:
    a. certain drugs
    b. chemical processes
    c. surgical hair transplantation
    d. scalp reduction
    _____

139. Which of the following is not considered a type of surgical hair restoration?
    a. flap surgery
    b. knotting
    c. hair transplants
    d. scalp reduction
    _____

140. What is the first step in cleaning a ready-made wig?
    a. Brush to remove surface dirt
    b. Rinse the wig in cold water
    c. Pin the wig to a head mold
    d. Dip the wig into wig solution
    _____

141. The process used to chemically restructure straight hair into a wave pattern is:
    a. permanent waving
    b. haircoloring
    c. reformation curls
    d. hair relaxing
    _____

142. A soft-curl perm is also known as all of the following *except* a:
    a. chemical blow-out
    b. Jheri curl
    c. reformation curl
    d. curl
    _____

143. The process used to rearrange over-curly hair into a straightened hair form is known as:
    a. a permanent wave
    b. a curl
    c. a reformation curl
    d. chemical hair relaxing
    _____

144. The two layers of the hair most affected by chemical texture services are the:
    a. cortex and medulla
    b. cortex and cuticle
    c. medulla and cuticle
    d. cortex and hair root _____

145. The partial or total removal of natural pigment or artificial color from the hair is called:
    a. hair lightening
    b. hair stripping
    c. haircoloring
    d. hair dying _____

146. The four classifications of haircoloring products include temporary and all of the following *except:*
    a. semipermanent
    b. permanent
    c. demipermanent
    d. temporary semipermanent _____

147. Temporary haircolor products are a type of:
    a. oxidation color
    b. penetrating color
    c. nonoxidation color
    d. self-penetrating color _____

148. Characteristics of permanent haircolor products include the following *except* that they:
    a. are mixed with hydrogen peroxide
    b. do not need retouch applications
    c. deposit and lift
    d. are penetrating tints _____

149. The technical term applied to any deformity or disease of the nail is:
    a. onychosis
    b. melanonychia
    c. eponychium
    d. leukonychia _____

150. Business operating expenses are also known as:
    a. overhead
    b. accounts receivables
    c. credits
    d. tax rebates _____

Answers to Chapter Review Tests

CHAPTER 1

1. a	2. a	3. c	4. d	5. b
6. a	7. c	8. a	9. d	10. b
11. d	12. a	13. b	14. c	15. d
16. b	17. a	18. c	19. d	

CHAPTER 2

1. c	2. c	3. c	4. a	5. d
6. b	7. c	8. a	9. b	10. c
11. d	12. c	13. c	14. a	15. c
16. b	17. a	18. d	19. a	20. c

CHAPTER 3

1. c	2. a	3. c	4. b	5. b
6. b	7. a	8. b	9. d	10. a
11. c	12. d	13. d	14. d	15. b
16. c	17. d	18. c	19. d	20. a
21. c	22. a	23. d	24. c	25. a
26. a	27. c	28. c	29. a	30. c
31. b	32. a	33. a	34. b	35. b

CHAPTER 4

1. c	2. c	3. b	4. c	5. b
6. b	7. a	8. c	9. b	10. d
11. b	12. d	13. a	14. c	15. d
16. a	17. a	18. b	19. b	20. a
21. d	22. c	23. c	24. d	25. a
26. d	27. b	28. b	29. a	30. a
31. d	32. c	33. d	34. a	35. b
36. a				

CHAPTER 5

1. c	2. b	3. d	4. d	5. c
6. a	7. b	8. b	9. d	10. c
11. a	12. c	13. b	14. a	15. c
16. a	17. b	18. d	19. d	20. b
21. d	22. d	23. a	24. b	25. a
26. b	27. b	28. a	29. b	30. a
31. a	32. a	33. a	34. c	35. c
36. a	37. b	38. a	39. c	40. c
41. d	42. a	43. a	44. d	45. d
46. a	47. a	48. d	49. c	50. a
51. a				

CHAPTER 6

1. c	2. b	3. d	4. b	5. d
6. c	7. d	8. a	9. c	10. d
11. c	12. a	13. b	14. a	15. a
16. a	17. d	18. a	19. a	20. a
21. d	22. a	23. b	24. c	25. a
26. b	27. c	28. d	29. d	30. d
31. a	32. b	33. d	34. b	35. b
36. c	37. a	38. b	39. c	40. a
41. d	42. b	43. a	44. c	45. d
46. a	47. b	48. a	49. d	50. b

CHAPTER 7

1. a	2. d	3. d	4. d	5. a
6. c	7. b	8. a	9. b	10. d
11. c	12. c	13. d	14. b	15. a
16. b	17. a	18. c	19. b	20. a
21. d	22. b	23. b	24. a	25. b
26. d	27. a	28. b	29. b	30. b

31. a	32. a	33. a	34. b	35. c
36. d	37. c	38. d	39. c	40. d
41. b	42. a	43. c	44. c	45. a
46. c	47. b	48. d	49. c	50. a
51. a	52. a	53. d	54. c	55. c
56. a	57. c	58. c	59. a	60. b
61. b	62. c	63. a	64. a	

CHAPTER 8

1. d	2. a	3. b	4. d	5. b
6. d	7. a	8. d	9. c	10. a
11. b	12. d	13. a	14. c	15. b
16. a	17. b	18. c	19. a	20. c
21. a	22. b	23. b	24. d	25. a
26. b	27. d	28. d	29. c	30. a
31. a	32. a	33. b	34. c	35. d
36. c	37. a	38. b	39. d	40. c
41. a	42. a	43. d	44. d	45. b
46. d	47. d	48. d		

CHAPTER 9

1. b	2. a	3. b	4. c	5. c
6. a	7. b	8. c	9. a	10. c
11. a	12. c	13. b	14. c	15. c
16. d	17. d	18. c	19. a	20. b
21. d	22. b	23. c	24. b	25. c
26. c	27. c	28. b	29. b	30. c

CHAPTER 10

1. d	2. a	3. c	4. d	5. a
6. c	7. b	8. d	9. b	10. d
11. d	12. c	13. c	14. b	15. a

16. a	17. b	18. c	19. b	20. a
21. b	22. a	23. b	24. c	25. a
26. a	27. d	28. b	29. d	30. a
31. d	32. a	33. c	34. a	35. d
36. d	37. b	38. b	39. c	40. b
41. a	42. c	43. a	44. c	45. b
46. a	47. c	48. b	49. d	50. b
51. c	52. d	53. b	54. d	55. c
56. a	57. a	58. d	59. b	60. b
61. c	62. d			

CHAPTER 11

1. a	2. a	3. a	4. b	5. c
6. b	7. a	8. c	9. c	10. a
11. c	12. b	13. c	14. d	15. a
16. a	17. b	18. b	19. a	20. c
21. a	22. b	23. b	24. d	25. a
26. c	27. d	28. c	29. b	30. b
31. c	32. d	33. a	34. a	35. c
36. a	37. c	38. d	39. a	40. c
41. a	42. b	43. c	44. a	45. d
46. c	47. c	48. d	49. b	50. a
51. a	52. c	53. d	54. c	55. b
56. a	57. b	58. b	59. a	60. c
61. b	62. a	63. d	64. c	65. c
66. a	67. a	68. c	69. d	70. d
71. b				

CHAPTER 12

| 1. d | 2. a | 3. c | 4. d | 5. a |
| 6. b | 7. c | 8. b | 9. c | 10. d |

11. d	12. a	13. a	14. h	15. b
16. a	17. b	18. a	19. c	20. b
21. a	22. c	23. d	24. c	25. b
26. d	27. b	28. a		

CHAPTER 13

1. d	2. d	3. b	4. d	5. d
6. a	7. b	8. a	9. b	10. d
11. b	12. a	13. c	14. d	15. b
16. d	17. a	18. a	19. c	20. a
21. a	22. c	23. b	24. d	25. b
26. d	27. b	28. c	29. c	30. a
31. d	32. a	33. c	34. c	35. b
36. b	37. a	38. d	39. d	40. a
41. c	42. a	43. d	44. a	45. c
46. b	47. c	48. a	49. a	50. a
51. c	52. b	53. c	54. a	55. c
56. a	57. c	58. c	59. b	60. d
61. c	62. c	63. a	64. a	65. c
66. d	67. c	68. d	69. c	70. b
71. a	72. d	73. b	74. d	75. a
76. c	77. d	78. a		

CHAPTER 14

1. a	2. b	3. b	4. c	5. c
6. c	7. c	8. c	9. d	10. c
11. b	12. b	13. b	14. c	15. a
16. c	17. b	18. b	19. c	20. a
21. a	22. d	23. a	24. c	25. d
26. a	27. c	28. c	29. a	30. a
31. c	32. d	33. b	34. a	35. c

36. b	37. d	38. d	39. c	40. c
41. c	42. c	43. d	44. a	45. c
46. a	47. a			

CHAPTER 15

1. a	2. c	3. b	4. b	5. a
6. b	7. c	8. a	9. d	10. d
11. d	12. a	13. c	14. b	15. d
16. b	17. a	18. b	19. c	20. a
21. c	22. b	23. a	24. b	25. d
26. b	27. d	28. d	29. d	30. b
31. d	32. b	33. b	34. c	35. d
36. c	37. a	38. c	39. b	40. a
41. a	42. a	43. d	44. d	45. a
46. b	47. a	48. d	49. b	50. b
51. c	52. d	53. a	54. a	55. b
56. d	57. b	58. c	59. d	60. b
61. c	62. c	63. a	64. a	65. b
66. c	67. a	68. b	69. c	

CHAPTER 16

1. d	2. a	3. b	4. d	5. d
6. b	7. b	8. d	9. a	10. c
11. b	12. d	13. b	14. b	15. a
16. c	17. c	18. c	19. d	20. a
21. b	22. c	23. a	24. b	25. b

CHAPTER 17

1. b	2. d	3. c	4. b	5. a
6. c	7. c	8. d	9. c	10. d
11. d	12. c	13. b	14. d	15. a

16. c	17. c	18. a	19. c	20. c
21. d	22. b	23. c	24. c	25. a
26. c				

CHAPTER 18

1. c	2. a	3. a	4. a	5. d
6. b	7. b	8. c	9. c	10. a
11. d	12. d	13. c	14. d	15. c
16. c	17. b	18. d	19. d	20. d
21. b	22. b	23. a	24. b	25. c
26. b	27. b	28. b	29. a	30. d
31. a	32. b	33. d	34. a	35. c
36. c	37. a	38. a	39. b	40. a
41. c	42. c	43. a	44. c	45. d
46. b	47. b	48. c	49. a	50. c
51. c	52. b	53. c	54. a	55. c
56. b	57. c	58. b	59. d	60. b
61. b	62. d	63. b	64. a	65. c
66. b	67. d	68. d	69. b	70. d

CHAPTER 19

1. d	2. b	3. a	4. d	5. b
6. d	7. c	8. d	9. a	10. a
11. c	12. a	13. a	14. b	15. a
16. d	17. a	18. c	19. b	20. b
21. c	22. d	23. d	24. b	25. c
26. a	27. c	28. a	29. a	30. d
31. a	32. a	33. a	34. d	35. b
36. d	37. d	38. c	39. d	40. b
41. a	42. a	43. c	44. b	45. c
46. a	47. d	48. b	49. c	50. b

51. b	52. d	53. d	54. c	55. a
56. b	57. d	58. c	59. d	60. a
61. c	62. c	63. b	64. c	65. c
66. a				

CHAPTER 20

1. a	2. d	3. c	4. a	5. c
6. d	7. b	8. d	9. c	10. b
11. d	12. b	13. a	14. d	15. a
16. c	17. d	18. b	19. d	20. b
21. b	22. c	23. d	24. a	25. c
26. d	27. c	28. d	29. a	30. c

CHAPTER 21

1. c	2. b	3. c	4. a	5. c
6. d	7. d	8. a	9. b	10. b
11. c	12. d	13. a	14. d	15. b
16. d	17. c	18. a	19. a	20. d

CHAPTER 22

1. a	2. d	3. d	4. c	5. c
6. c	7. a	8. a	9. d	10. d
11. a	12. b	13. d	14. d	15. c
16. c	17. a	18. a	19. a	20. b

CHAPTER 23

1. a	2. d	3. d	4. a	5. a
6. c	7. a	8. c	9. d	10. b
11. c	12. a	13. c	14. c	15. d
16. c	17. c	18. c	19. b	20. d
21. b	22. c	23. d	24. d	25. a
26. d				

Answers to Sample State Board Examinations

SAMPLE STATE BOARD EXAMINATION TEST 1

1. b	2. d	3. c	4. d	5. c
6. c	7. b	8. b	9. b	10. d
11. b	12. b	13. b	14. a	15. d
16. d	17. b.	18. a	19. c	20. a
21. a	22. c	23. d	24. d	25. c
26. c	27. b	28. c	29. d	30. b
31. c	32. c	33. a	34. b	35. a
36. b	37. d	38. c	39. a	40. b
41. a	42. c	43. b	44. b	45. d
46. b	47. a	48. d	49. c	50. d
51. b	52. a	53. c	54. d	55. c
56. b	57. c	58. a	59. a	60. d
61. b	62. a	63. d	64. b	65. a
66. c	67. a	68. c	69. c	70. d
71. a	72. d	73. d	74. b	75. c
76. d	77. b	78. c	79. c	80. b
81. b	82. d	83. a	84. c	85. d
86. c	87. b	88. a	89. b	90. c
91. c	92. a	93. a	94. c	95. a
96. c	97. d	98. b	99. a	100. b
101. a	102. c	103. d	104. c	105. b
106. c	107. c	108. b	109. c	110. a
111. b	112. c	113. c	114. d	115. b
116. a	117. c	118. d	119. b	120. d
121. a	122. b	123. a	124. d	125. b
126. b	127. b	128. a	129. a	130. d
131. a	132. d	133. d	134. b	135. b
136. b	137. c	138. b	139. b	140. a
141. a	142. a	143. d	144. b	145. a
146. d	147. c	148. b	149. b	150. a

SAMPLE STATE BOARD EXAMINATION TEST 2

1. b	2. d	3. d	4. c	5. b
6. b	7. b	8. a	9. c	10. d
11. b	12. b	13. b	14. a	15. d
16. d	17. b	18. a	19. c	20. a
21. a	22. c	23. d	24. d	25. c
26. c	27. b	28. c	29. d	30. b
31. c	32. c	33. a	34. d	35. a
36. c	37. d	38. d	39. a	40. b
41. a	42. c	43. b	44. c	45. d
46. b	47. b	48. d	49. b	50. d
51. b	52. a	53. d	54. d	55. c
56. b	57. c	58. b	59. a	60. d
61. b	62. a	63. d	64. b	65. a
66. c	67. a	68. c	69. c	70. d
71. a	72. d	73. d	74. c	75. b
76. d	77. b	78. c	79. c	80. b
81. b	82. d	83. a	84. c	85. d
86. a	87. b	88. a	89. b	90. c
91. c	92. c	93. a	94. a	95. a
96. c	97. c	98. b	99. a	100. b
101. a	102. c	103. d	104. c	105. b
106. c	107. c	108. b	109. a	110. a
111. c	112. c	113. c	114. d	115. b
116. a	117. c	118. d	119. d	120. d
121. a	122. b	123. a	124. d	125. b
126. b	127. a	128. b	129. c	130. d
131. a	132. d	133. d	134. b	135. b
136. b	137. c	138. b	139. b	140. a
141. a	142. a	143. d	144. b	145. a
146. d	147. c	148. b	149. a	150. a

SAMPLE STATE BOARD EXAMINATION TEST 3

1. a	2. d	3. d.	4. c	5. b
6. b	7. b	8. a	9. a	10. d
11. b	12. b	13. b	14. a	15. d
16. d	17. b	18. a	19. c	20. a
21. a	22. c	23. d	24. d	25. c
26. c	27. c	28. c	29. d	30. b
31. c	32. c	33. a	34. d	35. a
36. c	37. d	38. d	39. a	40. b
41. a	42. c	43. d	44. c	45. d
46. b	47. b	48. d	49. b	50. d
51. b	52. a	53. d	54. d	55. c
56. b	57. c	58. b	59. a	60. d
61. b	62. a	63. d	64. b	65. a
66. c	67. a	68. c	69. c	70. d
71. a	72. d	73. d	74. c	75. c
76. d	77. b	78. c	79. c	80. b
81. b	82. d	83. a	84. c	85. d
86. a	87. b	88. c	89. b	90. c
91. c	92. c	93. a	94. a	95. a
96. c	97. c	98. b	99. a	100. b
101. a	102. c	103. d	104. c	105. b
106. c	107. c	108. b	109. a	110. a
111. c	112. c	113. c	114. d	115. b
116. a	117. c	118. d	119. d	120. d
121. a	122. c	123. b	124. d	125. b
126. b	127. a	128. b	129. c	130. d
131. a	132. d	133. d	134. b	135. b
136. b	137. c	138. b	139. b	140. a
141. a	142. a	143. d	144. b	145. a
146. d	147. c	148. b	149. a	150. a

PART III—Helpful Reminders for Examination Day

The following reminders have been prepared for your benefit and will assist you in passing the state board examinations.

1. *Take the time to present a professional appearance.* This includes your clothing, personal hygiene, general health, and posture.

2. *Adopt a positive mental attitude.* Doing so will help you to overcome the nervousness often associated with taking test and exams. It might help to remember that state board exams are not given to make candidates fail, but to do justice to all candidates by using measurable and objective methods of evaluation. Testing and evaluation are vital to determining a candidate's competency for the profession.

3. *Be prepared.* Create a checklist of the supplies and tools you will need for both exams. Be guided by the candidate information that usually accompanies confirmation of the test date. Make sure you bring a photo ID for identification purposes.

4. *Be punctual.* Learn in advance how to reach the test site and allow sufficient time for travel. Being on time for the exam will alleviate some stress and make it easier to maintain a positive attitude so that you can do your best.

5. *Written or computer-based tests.* Some general reminders for written or computer-based testing include the following:
   - Be ready to begin when the signal is given by the test proctor.
   - Scan the entire test before beginning to answer the questions. Then read each test item carefully and answer the questions consecutively whenever possible.
   - Avoid spending too much time on one test item; if in doubt, continue with the test and return to the unanswered item(s) after completing the entire test.
   - If time permits, review all your answers before submitting the completed test.

6. *Practical exams.* General reminders for practical exams include:
   - Ask questions of the examiner before the signal to begin is given. Talking is prohibited during the exam.
   - Observe all sanitation rules during the practical exam. The use of proper cleaning methods is vital to a passing score.
   - Use only clean tools and implements.
   - Wash your hands before beginning each service.
   - Make sure your model is draped correctly for each service.
   - Do not put combs or implements in pockets.
   - Do not set a tool or implement down and reuse it without cleaning it first.